SUGAR
COUNTER

SUGAR COUNTER
for health

The Smart Person's Guide to Hidden Sugars

Dr Elizabeth Roberts

SOUVENIR PRESS

First published in Great Britain in 2016 by Souvenir Press Ltd
43 Great Russell Street, London WC1B 3PD

ISBN 9780285643291

Typeset by M Rules
Printed and bound in Denmark by Nørhaven

CONTENTS

Author's Introduction	vii
Alcoholic drinks	1
Beans and Pulses	5
Biscuits and Crackers	9
Breads, pastry, flour and baked goods	13
Cakes and pastries	21
Cooked dishes containing meat and poultry	27
Cooking and baking ingredients, syrups and jams	35
Eggs and egg dishes	41
Fats and oils	43
Fish, fish dishes and seafood	49
Fruit – fresh, dried, stewed and tinned	59
Grains and cereals	71
Herbs and spices	77
Meat and meat products	79
Milk and dairy products	85
Non-alcoholic drinks and beverages	95
Nuts and seeds	103
Potatoes and potato dishes	107
Poultry	111
Puddings and ice-cream	115
Rice, noodles and pasta	123

Salads and light meals   129

Sauces and condiments   137

Snacks, dips and crisps   145

Soups and sandwiches   149

Sweets and confectionary   153

Takeaway food   157

Vegetables and vegetable dishes   163

Vegetarian dishes   177

Vegetarian meat alternatives   187

Introduction

It wasn't so long ago that a merry jingle told us how 'a Mars a day helps you work rest and play'.

Taken to heart, that would mean a sugar intake of 10.7 teaspoons a day – around 75 teaspoons a week, according to figures from the British Dental Foundation. Glug a daily can of CocaCola, another 8.1 teaspoons a day, or 56.7 a week, and you've a daily sugar consumption of 18.8 teaspoons – before you've added breakfast cereal, toast, pizza, chicken in BBQ sauce, a banana, yogurt, a glass of wine, all of them containing sugar. And do you put sugar in your tea and coffee?

The World Health Organisation recommends that we consume no more than 6 teaspoons of sugar a day. Many of us – the majority of us – are consuming many more than that. In so doing, we are setting ourselves up for innumerable long-term and serious health problems.

One in four Britons is obese, according to the UN Food and Agriculture Organisation. Britain has the highest levels of obesity in Western Europe.

And the root cause? Sugar.

Jamie Oliver, chef, author and food and health campaigner, likes to talk about 'honest' and 'dishonest' sugars. The former are those we *know* we are ingesting – in that bar of chocolate perhaps, or a coffee. The latter – often disguised under another name – are the hidden sugars that occur in foods. Savoury foods, where we might not expect to find sugar – tomato soup, a pizza, BBQ sauce for example. Low-fat foods, where added sugar is used to enhance flavour and texture.

Fizzy drinks are a particular problem, for many of us are unaware just *how* much sugar they contain. Jamie Oliver is advocating a tax on them, with the money raised being put to good use – primary schools and the NHS. He has set an example by levying a tax on drinks with added sugar in his own restaurants. He and others want to see far more government regulation of the food and drinks industry, making manufacturers come clean about hidden sugars and much besides. Sadly the government seems to prefer self-regulation and industry-funded research designed to obscure rather than clarify.

As a dietitian, I know only too well how difficult it can be for people to make sense of food labels. Looking through food labels with clients is often a revelation, especially when people are making choices they think are healthy. A family history of breast cancer led me to conduct my own research into what constitutes a truly healthy diet, beyond the advice I was taught to give out as a dietitian. And the first change that I made to my own diet? To cut right down on sugar. I soon realised what a minefield food labelling can be and so decided to write this book to help consumers navigate the food aisles.

The *Sugar Counter for Health* will help you decode the labels on every-day foods and ingredients, enabling you to know exactly what you're buying and what you're eating.

The scale of the problem

The dangers of eating too much are now increasingly clear. Levels of consumption once considered safe are now known to be unsafe and official bodies are revising their guidelines. Added sugar – contained in so many everyday foods – is a particular hazard. Often we're not even aware that we are eating it and that of course makes it all too easy to eat more than we should.

The World Health Organisation (WHO) suggested recently that less than 5% of our total daily calorie intake be added sugar – a halving of its previous recommendation of no more than 10%.

In the UK, the Scientific Advisory Committee for Nutrition (SACN) has been even more radical. It too now recommends a daily 5% maximum. But until recently SACN had been happy that added sugar form as much as 11–15% of daily calorie intake.

Added sugar is defined as sugars that are 'added to foods by the manufacturer, cook, or consumer, plus sugars naturally present in honey, syrups, and fruit juices'

So how can we know how much sugar we are eating?

It's easy to know the total sugar content of packaged foods: the law requires that it be stated on the food label. It is trickier for foods that are not labelled – for example, foods we have prepared ourselves.

There are different types of sugars and these can be either naturally occurring or added to food. Although food labels tell us how much total sugar is contained in a particular food, they tell us nothing about the *type* of sugar. Not all sugars are thought to be harmful – the sugars found naturally in fresh milk, for example. Neither do food labels tell us whether sugar is added or naturally occurring. Naturally occurring sugars – such as those in fresh fruit – are not thought to be so harmful because the sugar comes 'attached' to the natural fibre in the food, lessening its negative impact on our bodies. People can find this confusing and worry unnecessarily about naturally occurring sugars.

Despite the dangers of too much added sugar, food manufacturers are still not required to tell us how much they add to our food. The *Sugar Counter for Health* uses the latest national food analysis in the UK as a guide to the sugars that are hidden in our food. As well as the amount of total sugar, it details the amount of sucrose, fructose and glucose contained in more than 2,500 foods and drinks. By checking the amount of each, you will understand how much sugar can be hidden in your everyday foods.

How to use this sugar guide

You can use *The Sugar Counter for Health* simply to check the total sugar content of most of your everyday foods, including cooked foods and meals. However, it doesn't reveal the whole picture. Some of the total sugar may be comprised of different types of sugar that aren't unhealthy. Take milk: whole milk contains 4.8g of sugar per 100g, and yet it contains no fructose or sucrose. This is because all the 'sugar' in milk is in the form of milk sugar, or lactose. Lactose is not thought to contribute to obesity, diabetes and other metabolic disorders.

You might want to go one step further and use this guide to check out the sucrose, fructose and glucose content of the foods you eat in order to form an idea of whether sugar might be added. Although food manufacturers may add sugar in the form of sugar syrups which contain varying amounts of glucose, fructose and other sugars, sucrose is found in food mainly when it is added. The exception to this is fresh, whole fruit. Peaches for example contain 5.2g of sucrose per 100g. As these are raw, unprocessed peaches, all this sucrose will be naturally occurring.

Now look at 'Muffins, American, not chocolate'. See all that sucrose (24.3g)? That will be added to the muffins as table sugar in food processing. Large amounts of glucose suggest that this too may have been added. Excess fructose is thought to be the main reason that sugar leads to health problems.

For each food item included in this guide, the food is listed per 100g as weighed. For some items, the food is listed twice – weighed before *and* after preparation. For example, under 'Fish, fish dishes and seafood' you will find that lobster is listed twice: Lobster, boiled and Lobster, boiled, weighed with shell. The first should be used if you cook the lobster and then remove the shell before weighing. You should use the second if you weighed the lobster before removing the shell. Some foods include both a raw and a cooked weight, depending on whether or not you weighed the food before cooking – these foods will lose weight during cooking, mainly from water loss.

The information about total sugar, sucrose, fructose and glucose in this guide is sourced from the UK Composition of Foods Integrated Dataset (CoFID), a national project to analyse foods commonly consumed in the UK. The information was updated in 2015, when most foods were re-analysed to reflect recent changes in food composition by manufacturers. For each food item, the amount of total sugars and teaspoons (tsp) of sugar per 100g and per portion size is given, as well as the amount of sucrose, fructose and glucose per 100g. Teaspoons of sugar are rounded to the nearest quarter teaspoon. Where the letter N appears instead of a value, this means that the amount of sucrose, fructose and/or glucose for this particular food was not analysed by CoFID. 'Tr' stands for Trace – meaning there was a little of the particular sugar, but less than 0.1g per 100g.

Portion sizes were calculated from the Food Standards Agency's *Food Portion Sizes* (3rd edition) and manufacturer labelling. Do check the serving size of the brand you eat though – there is little consistency in food portion sizes. For vegetables, Public Health England's 5-a-Day portion sizes was also used. For some foods used as ingredients, such as flour, we have not included a portion size. Instead, we have used a 28g (10oz) serving for guidance.

What exactly is sugar?

The energy (calories) we get from food can come from alcohol, fat, protein and from carbohydrates. Carbohydrates come from both starch and from sugars. There are many different types of sugars and several different chemical compounds that are classed as 'sugars'. Only two – glucose and fructose – have been associated with obesity, diabetes, gout and blood lipid disorders. The compound we refer to as 'sugar' is called sucrose by scientists and dietitians. It actually consists of two molecules bound together – one of glucose and one of fructose. Each of these molecules cause their own problems, which is why added sugar is so bad for us – you get two lots of problems in one go.

What is the problem with sugar?

The problems with sugar come from both the glucose and the fructose molecule. Glucose stimulates the production of insulin by our pancreas. Insulin is a hormone that regulates our blood sugar (glucose) levels. All starchy foods are made up of chains of glucose which are broken down into single glucose molecules through our digestion. When glucose occurs naturally in foods, it is usually bound up ('stuck') to the cell wall of the plant, as in the case of whole fruits and whole grains. This means it takes our bodies longer to break down the food and extract the glucose. The glucose is released more slowly into our bloodstream, over several hours, and so our pancreas needs to make less insulin. One of the problems with sugar is that the glucose is released very quickly, causing a spike in insulin pro-duction to counteract this.

This is particularly harmful when glucose occurs in drinks. Liquids are absorbed more quickly from our stomachs than solid food. Thus, the glucose enters our bloodstream even more quickly. This explains the focus on the sugar in fruit juice and fizzy drinks.

The other problem with sugar, or sucrose, is the fructose molecule. We can only metabolise small amounts of fructose at a time, and mainly in our livers. Some argue that this is because we never evolved to consume large amounts of fructose. In nature, fructose exists only in small amounts in fruit, honey and other natural syrups. It is thought that fructose causes resistance to the effects of insulin in our liver and muscles. As our bodies become more and more resistant to insulin for processing glucose, our pancreas has to produce even more insulin to clear glucose from our blood stream.

How much sugar can I eat?

As we've seen, official bodies once recommended that we consume no more than 10% of our total daily calorie (kcal) intake as added sugar. Public Health England is responsible for surveying the nation's dietary habits. The 2008–2012 National Diet and Nutrition Survey found that all age groups consume well in excess of this 10% guideline. Children aged between 4 and 10 consume around 14.7% of their kcal intake as added sugar. For 11 to 18 year-olds, added sugar accounts for 15.4% of kcal intake. For adults aged between 19 and 64, the figure is 11.5%. The amount of sugar that children are consuming is particularly worrying, given the rising levels of obesity in children. Linked to this, an ever greater number of children in the UK are being diagnosed with diabetes than ever before.

As the evidence about the dangers of too much sugar in our diets continues to grow, recommendations are being revised downwards. Both the World Health Organisation and the UK Scientific Advisory Committee on Nutrition now recommend that we consume no more than 5% of our daily calorie requirements in the form of added sugar.

Calorie requirements will of course depend on our activity levels, but for an average man it is somewhere in the region of 2,500 kcal per day and for an average woman around 2,000 kcal. This means no more than 31.25g, or 7.8 teaspoons (tsp), of added sugar each day for the average man and

25g, and 6.25 teaspoons for the average woman. Each g of sugar has roughly 4 kcal.

The table below details how much sugar is acceptable for different daily calorie (kcal) intakes. Remember, this isn't your *total* sugar allowance, but rather how much *added* sugar it is OK to have. Therefore, it does not include the sugar in milk or fresh fruit, but it does include the sugar in fruit juice.

Daily calorie (kcal) intake	Added sugar allowance as 5% of kcal	Added sugar allowance in grams (g)	Added sugar allowance in teaspoon (tsp)
1,600	80	20	5
1,700	85	21.25	5.3
1,800	90	22.5	5.6
1,900	95	23.75	5.9
2,000	100	25	6.25
2,100	105	26.25	6.6
2,200	110	27.5	6.9
2,300	115	28.75	7.2
2,400	120	30	7.5
2,500	125	31.25	7.8
2,600	130	32.5	8.1
2,700	135	33.75	8.4
2,800	140	35	8.75

A typical breakfast consisting of a medium slice of brown toast and jam, and a small 35g serving of bran flakes with milk, will provide 26.1g sugar. Add a BLT sandwich, a packet of crisps and a small carton of orange juice, and you are already up to 48.6g of sugar in total. With the exception of the sugar in the milk, and some of the naturally occurring sugars in the starchy foods, nearly all of this sugar is added. This is already well in excess of the 35g allowance for an active man who needs 2,800 kcal per day. And we haven't even added a pre-packaged pasta sauce for dinner and a sweet treat yet! To stick to the recommended intake, this same active man could switch to seeded bread for toast (1.4g per average slice) with spread and a boiled egg (just a trace of sugar). The same sandwich for lunch (4.7g), served with a small bag of popped corn (0.5g) and a whole orange (11.6g) would bring his total sugar intake down to 18.2g, be much healthier and leave room for a sweet treat.

How do I know how much sugar is in my food?

It is fairly easy to determine how much *total* sugar is in a food. Look for the 'Carbohydrates (of which sugars)' figure in the nutrition panel. A food that is high in sugar will have more than 22.5 g of total sugars per 100g. A food that is low in total sugars will have 5g or less of total sugars per 100g. If the amount of sugars per 100g is between these two figures, then it has a medium level of total sugars. In the sample nutrition panel below, this food is (just) high in total sugars.

A word of caution: all foods must declare their nutritional content per 100g (or per 100ml for drinks). Many will also give values per serving size. Be careful when using serving size: the manufacturer decides what this is, and it may not be the same as your own serving size!

Table of Nutritional Information		
	Per 100g	*Per 45g*
Energy	1760 kJ 418 kcal	792 kJ 188 kcal
Fat	9.2g	0.6g
of which saturates	1.2g	0.6g
Carbohydrate	70.9g	31.9g
of which sugars	22.5g	10.1g
Fibre	6.8g	3.1g
Protein	8.0g	3.6g
Salt	0.01g	0.01g

Deciphering how much sugar is added to food is a whole other story – and virtually impossible. When food is analysed in a lab, the lab cannot tell whether a particular type of sugar is added or occurs naturally in the food. Manufacturers claim they cannot tell us how much sugar they add to foods as this would give away the recipes to their competitors. As yet, no government has compelled manufacturers to declare how much sugar is added to food. Given the power and influence of the food industry, we may be waiting for some time yet.

As it's not possible to identify added from naturally occurring sugar, the best way to gauge whether the total sugar in a food is added is to read the ingredients list which details all the ingredients in a food in descending order of weight. Thus, the ingredient of which there is most will appear first in the list, the second largest ingredient second. And so forth. This is why ingredients such as additives usually appear towards the end of the list – gram for gram there is less of them than of the other ingredients.

One way in which manufacturers can 'hide' the amount of added sugar in food is to use different types of sugars instead of just one. In this way, less of each is needed, and so each type appears lower down the list of ingredients. This might give the consumer the false impression that the food contains less sugar than is actually the case. The savvy shopper should look for the following words on the list of ingredients that may be used to describe the different types of added sugars:

agave nectar	brown sugar	cane sugar or cane syrup	coconut sugar
concentrated fruit juice	corn syrup	dextrose	fructose
fruit sugar	glucose	glucose syrup	glucose–fructose syrup
grape sugar	honey	hydrolysed starch	invert(ed) sugar
maltodextrin	maltose	malt syrup	maple syrup
molasses	palm sugar	sucrose	syrup

Although honey, agave nectar and maple syrup are marketed in many sugar-free foods and recipes as healthier alternatives to sugar, they're really just other forms of sugar, and have the same effect on the body. In the sample ingredients list below, see if you can spot any hidden sugars.

Ingredients

Rolled Oats (54%), Sugar, Glucose Syrup, Raisins (10%), Sunflower Oil, Cereal Crisps (Rice Flour, Wheat Flour), Humectant: Glycerol, Oat Bran,

Honey, Colour (Plain Caramel), Natural Raisin Flavouring, Antioxidant (Tocopherol)

In this food, sugar has been added as three separate ingredients: plain sugar, glucose syrup and honey. This gives the impression that the food has less sugar than it really does, as each type of sugar accounts for a small amount of the total sugar. Add them up though, and that amounts to a lot of sugar.

Sugar and weight gain

Traditional dietary guidelines assert that burning more calories than we take in is all that matters if we want to lose weight. This way of thinking is being questioned. We now believe that calories from different sources (called 'macronutrients' by scientists and dietitians) are metabolised differently in our bodies. That means calories from different macronutrients have very different effects on how we store energy, and on our appetite.

When we eat large amounts of glucose, either from sugar or from refined starchy foods, our body is subjected to a rush of glucose. This is particularly problematic when we eat foods without fibre, such as white rice, bread and pasta. This is because fibre can help slow down the speed at which the food leaves our stomach and how quickly it enters our bloodstream. This surge of insulin encourages fat storage. When our insulin levels are constantly high (known as hyperinsulinaemia), the hormones that regulate our appetite are disrupted. This can then make us feel hungrier, causing us to overeat and never quite feel full. As we become resistant to the effects of insulin, our system has to make larger and larger amounts of it whenever we eat carbohydrate. This is a recipe for weight gain, especially around the middle, when it is known as central adiposity.

Sugar and diabetes

There are two types of diabetes, known as Type 1 and Type 2.

Type 1 is the rarer of the two and it usually occurs suddenly, and at a younger age. The cause is thought to be an autoimmune reaction in which the body attacks itself. The cells in the pancreas that produce insulin are destroyed and the person then has to inject insulin for the rest of their lives.

Type 2 is the second and more common form. People with Type 2 diabetes do not usually have to inject insulin, at least not in the beginning. When you hear about the 'diabetes epidemic', it is Type 2 that we are referring to. Type 2 diabetes usually occurs later in life and is therefore often referred to as late onset diabetes. In contrast to Type 1 diabetes, Type 2 diabetes is almost entirely down to our lifestyles. Our genetic make-up may play some part, but the disease was almost non-existent before the introduction of Western diets.

Many authorities maintain that sugar has no direct effect on the diabetes epidemic. They say sugar only contributes to the development of diabetes by adding extra 'empty' calories to our diet. They say that it is these empty calories that cause weight gain and that it is the *weight gain itself* that causes diabetes, rather than any specific effect of the sugar. Nevertheless, many researchers are now suggesting that sugar, and particularly *added* sugar, may have a direct effect on causing diabetes. A constant onslaught of glucose, consumed through sugar and refined carbohydrates, forces the pancreas to produce more insulin. Added to this is resistance to the effects of insulin from the fructose in sugar. All in all, the perfect recipe for an over-worked pancreas.

Whatever the role of sugar in causing Type 2 diabetes, reducing your sugar intake, particularly from added sugars, is likely to lower your risk of developing the disease. If you already have diabetes, all is not lost: eating less sugar and refined carbohydrates should improve your blood sugar (glucose) control.

Sugar and the risk of cancer

It is increasingly thought that hyperinsulinaemia, or persistently raised insulin levels, contributes to the development of certain 'environmental' cancers. This includes, for example, breast cancer and colorectal cancer. Insulin acts as a growth hormone and it is thought that insulin can trigger, or accelerate, the growth of malignant cancer cells. Central adiposity, or belly fat, produces chemicals that can cause inflammation. These chemicals are also thought to trigger cancer cell growth. Although there are many aspects of our modern diets that contribute to our risk of some cancers, reducing sugar intake will be a step in the right direction.

Sugar, blood lipid disorders and heart disease

Traditional thinking has been that eating fat, particularly saturated fat, raises blood cholesterol levels. Raised cholesterol in turn may cause heart disease by clogging our arteries. Too much salt raises our blood pressure, and raised blood pressure can make the walls of the arteries thicker.

More recent thinking considers the role of insulin, sugar and refined carbohydrates in the development of cardiovascular disease. As previously mentioned, insulin acts as a growth hormone. It is thought that hyperinsulinaemia can cause growth and thickening of the arterial walls which in turn raises blood pressure. One of the by-products of sugar metabolism in the liver is a chemical that raises blood pressure. Chemicals made in our belly fat cause inflammation, scarring and the deposit of bad fats in the arterial walls.

Cholesterol is just part of the vehicle for carrying different types of fats in our bloodstream. The vehicle itself is known as a lipoprotein. Lipoproteins carry cholesterol and fats around our bodies. Cholesterol is an important building block for many hormones and other functions in our bodies. Lipoproteins carry fats from the liver to fat cells for storage when we have taken in more calories than we need, or back to the liver to make glucose when we haven't eaten for a while. The fats carried by the lipoproteins are called triglycerides.

Cholesterol was used as a measure in the early days of research into heart disease because it was the only thing that could be easily measured. Lots of cholesterol means lots of lipoproteins. We now know that cholesterol, or rather the lipoproteins, transports fats differently. Most people have heard about 'good' and 'bad' cholesterol but it's actually a misnomer: the cholesterol is exactly the same in both. It is the entire lipoprotein, and the cholesterol and fats it carries, that is good or bad.

Although saturated fat does indeed raise the number of lipoproteins and therefore the amount of total cholesterol, we now know that there are different types of lipoproteins. We probably all know that High Density Lipoproteins (HDL) are good. Traditionally, we have thought that Low Density Lipoproteins (LDL) were bad. We have recently discovered that there are two different types of LDL – small, dense particles and lighter, fluffier particles. The small dense particles are indeed bad, as they burrow into the walls of our arteries and cause fatty deposits. The lighter, fluffier ones do not – but both are counted together when we talk about 'bad' LDL cholesterol. You won't know exactly how much of each type you have. We now believe that the smaller, denser LDL particles come from Very Low Density Lipoproteins (VLDL). And where does much of our VLDL come from? Yep, you guessed it: fructose and excess carbohydrates. **Our low–fat craze has meant that we are eating more sugar and refined carbohydrates than ever before. Food manufacturers often replace the fat that is taken out of food with sugar or sweeteners for flavour, and starches for thickness and 'mouthfeel'.**

Sugar and gout

Gout often appears alongside other signs of 'metabolic' disorder, such as obesity, Type 2 diabetes, high blood pressure and blood lipid disorders. Gout was traditionally thought of as a disease of excess for it often attacked more affluent and 'portly' gentlemen partial to eating lots of meat and drinking plenty of alcohol.

Traditional dietary advice focused on reducing purines in the diet. Purines are a type of amino acid that makes up proteins. Purines are broken down to another compound called uric acid. Increased levels of uric acid are a feature of gout. But guess what? So is sugar. Recent research has shown that some fructose is turned into uric acid in our livers. A century ago, more affluent men (and women) did indeed consume more meat than poorer people – but they also consumed more sugar, then a luxury item locked away from the servants.

Why do we use so much sugar?

Food manufacturers add sugar to our food for many reasons, but mainly because we like the taste! Sugar can make cheap and poor ingredients taste better. Sugar can be used as a preservative. It also helps to brown certain foods, like baked bread. Along with other added ingredients it can improve moisture retention, keeping bread, cakes and doughnuts softer for longer. It is also cheap, which is the main reason the volume of sugar we consume has skyrocketed.

In the 1700s we were eating around 1.8kg (4lbs) of sugar each per year. By the 1800s, this had risen to 8.2kg (18lbs) and it continued to rise. Although sugar consumption is falling again, we are still eating a whopping 30kg (66lbs) each per year. And although in Britain we are now eating less table sugar, we are consuming more sugar through processed foods. Our bodies were never designed to metabolise this amount of sugar which is why it causes so many problems.

Our knowledge of the health problems that too much sugar causes continues to mount. From obesity and diabetes, to gout and heart disease; the list keeps growing. Some say it might even be addictive. Whether this is true or not, we just can't get enough of the sweet stuff. And food manufacturers know it. A careful look at food labels and *The Sugar Counter for Health* will arm you with the tools you need to take control of your sugar intake. Get smart and uncover the hidden sugars.

Alcoholic drinks

You may notice that the ml and g in some
of the alcoholic drinks are different.
Although 1ml of water will always weigh 1g,
1 ml of other drinks can differ.
This depends on the "specific gravity"
of the drink.

Food name	Total sugars (g/100g)	Teaspoons (tsp) sugar/100g	Sucrose (g/100g)	Fructose (g/100g)	Glucose (g/100g)	Average portion size	Grams (g) sugar per average portion	Tsp sugar per average portion
Advocaat	28.4	7	26.7	0.0	1.7	1 measure – 25ml (27g)	7	1¾
Ale, pale, bottled	2.0	½	0.0	Tr	0.7	1 pint (574g)	11.5	3
						½ pint (287g)	5.7	1½
						500 ml bottle or can (501g)	10.0	2½
						440 ml can (441g)	8.8	2¼
						275ml bottle (276g)	5.5	1½
Ale, strong ale/barley wine	6.1	1½	0.0	Tr	Tr	1 pint (574g)	35.0	8¾
						½ pint (287g)	17.5	4
						500 ml bottle or can (509g)	31.0	7¾
						440 ml can (448g)	27.3	6¾
						275ml bottle (280g)	17.1	4¼
Beer, bitter, average (<4% ABV)	2.2	½	0.0	0.0	0.0	1 pint (574g)	12.6	3¼
						½ pint (287g)	6.3	1½
						500 ml bottle or can (504g)	11.1	2¾
						440 ml can (443g)	9.7	2
						275ml bottle (277g)	6.1	1½
Beer, bitter, best, premium	2.2	½	0.0	0.0	0.3	1 pint (574g)	12.6	3¼
						½ pint (287g)	6.3	1½
						500 ml bottle or can (504g)	11.1	2¾
						440 ml can (443g)	9.7	2½
						275ml bottle (277g)	6.1	1½
Beer, bitter, low alcohol	1.2	½	0.0	0.1	0.4	1 pint (574g)	6.9	1¾
						½ pint (287g)	3.4	¾
						500 ml bottle or can (510g)	6.1	1½
						440 ml can (449g)	5.4	1¼
						275ml bottle (280g)	3.4	¾
Beer, bitter, strong (>5% ABV)	2.2	½	0.0	0.0	0.3	1 pint (574g)	12.6	3¼
						½ pint (287g)	6.3	1½
						500 ml bottle or can (500g)	11.0	2¾
						440 ml can (440g)	9.7	2½
						275ml bottle (275g)	6.1	1½
Beer, mild, draught	1.6	½	0.0	Tr	Tr	1 pint (574g)	9.2	2¼
						½ pint (287g)	4.6	1¼
						500 ml bottle or can (504g)	8.1	2
						440 ml can (444g)	7.1	1¾
						275ml bottle (277g)	4.4	1
Brown ale, bottled	3.0	¾	0.1	0.4	0.4	550 ml (554g)	16.6	4¼
Champagne	1.4	¼	Tr	0.8	0.6	1 glass – 150ml (149g)	2.1	½
Cider, dry	2.6	¾	0.7	0.5	0.6	1 pint 568ml (572g)	14.9	3¾
						½ pint 284ml (286g)	7.4	1¾
						500 ml bottle or can (503g)	13.1	3¼
						440ml can (443g)	11.5	3
Cider, low alcohol	3.6	1	1.4	1.4	0.7	1 pint 568ml (579g)	20.8	5¼
						½ pint 284ml (290g)	10.4	2½
						500 ml bottle or can (510g)	18.4	4½
						440ml can (449g)	16.2	4

Food name	Total sugars (g/100g)	Teaspoons (tsp) sugar/100g	Sucrose (g/100g)	Fructose (g/100g)	Glucose (g/100g)	Average portion size	Grams (g) sugar per average portion	Tsp sugar per average portion
Cider, strong	7.3	1¾	2.0	1.3	1.8	1 pint 568ml (578g)	42.2	10½
						½ pint 284ml (289g)	21.1	5¼
						500 ml bottle or can (508g)	37.1	9¼
						440ml can (447g)	32.6	8¼
Cider, sweet	4.3	1	1.2	0.7	1.0	1 pint 568ml (575g)	24.7	6¼
						½ pint 284ml (287g)	12.3	3
						500 ml bottle or can (506g)	21.8	5½
						440ml can (445g)	19.1	4¾
Coffee, Irish	2.5	¾	2.2	0.0	0.0	4 parts coffee, 2 parts whiskey, 1½ parts cream (140g)	3.5	1
Curacao	28.3	7				1 measure – 25 ml (26g)	7.4	1¾
Egg nog, homemade	9.6	2½	6.2	0.0	Tr	150 ml (164g)	15.7	4
Lager, alcohol-free	1.2	¼	Tr	0.4	0.6	1 pint (574g)	6.9	1¾
						½ pint (287g)	3.4	¾
						500 ml bottle or can (505g)	6.1	1½
						440 ml can (444g)	5.3	1¼
						275ml bottle (278g)	3.3	¾
Lager, extra strong	2.4	½	0.0	0.0	1.0	1 pint (574g)	13.8	3½
						½ pint (287g)	6.9	1¾
						500 ml bottle or can (502g)	12.0	3
						440 ml can (442g)	10.6	2¾
						275ml bottle (276g)	6.6	1¾
Lager, low alcohol	0.5	¼	0.0	0.1	0.3	1 pint (574g)	2.9	¾
						½ pint (287g)	1.4	¼
						500 ml bottle or can (505g)	2.5	¾
						440 ml can (444g)	2.2	½
						275ml bottle (278g)	1.4	¼
Lager, premium	Tr	0	0.0	0.0	Tr	1 pint (574g)	Tr	0
						½ pint (287g)	Tr	0
						500 ml bottle or can (502g)	Tr	0
						440 ml can (442g)	Tr	0
						275ml bottle (276g)	Tr	0
Lager, standard	Tr	0	0.0	0.0	Tr	1 pint (574g)	Tr	0
						½ pint (287g)	Tr	0
						500 ml bottle or can (502g)	Tr	0
						440 ml can (442g)	Tr	0
						275ml bottle (276g)	Tr	0
Liqueurs, cream (i.e. Baileys Original Irish Cream)	21.8	5½	21.0	0.0	0.0	1 measure – 25 ml (27g)	5.9	1½
Liqueurs, high strength (including Pernod, Drambuie, Cointreau, Grand Marnier and Southern Comfort)	24.4	6	17.1	2.3	2.6	1 measure – 25 ml (27g)	6.6	1¾

Food name	Total sugars (g/100g)	Teaspoons (tsp) sugar/100g	Sucrose (g/100g)	Fructose (g/100g)	Glucose (g/100g)	Average portion size	Grams (g) sugar per average portion	Tsp sugar per average portion
Liqueurs, low-medium strength (including cherry brandy, Tia Maria and Creme de Menthe)	32.8	8¼	20.4	6.1	6.3	1 measure – 25 ml (27g)	8.9	2¼
Port	12.0	3	2.8	4.6	4.6	1 small glass – 50ml (51g)	6.1	1½
Pre-mixed spirit based drinks (including WKD, Bacardi Breezer, Smirnoff Ice and Carribean Twist)	8.0	2	N	N	N	275ml (277g)	22.2	5½
Root beer	10.6	2½	N	N	N	375ml bottle (382g)	40.5	10¼
Shandy, 50% lager, homemade	2.9	¾	1.4	0.7	0.8	1 pint 568ml (579g)	16.8	4¼
						½ pint 284ml (278g)	8.1	2
Shandy, bottled or canned	5.0	1¼	1.7	1.7	1.6	330ml can (337g)	16.9	4¼
Sherry, dry	1.4	¼	0.0	0.7	0.7	1 small glass – 50ml (49g)	0.7	¼
Sherry, medium	5.9	1½	0.0	2.9	3.0	1 small glass – 50 ml (49g)	2.9	¾
Sherry, sweet	6.9	1¾	0.0	3.5	3.6	1 small glass – 50ml (50g)	3.5	1
Spirits, 40% volume	Tr	0	Tr	0.0	0.0	1 measure – 25ml (24g)	Tr	0
Stout, Mackeson	4.6	1¼	0.4	0.3	0.4	330 ml can (331g)	15.2	3¾
						275ml bottle (276g)	12.7	3¼
Stout, Guinness	3.2	¾	0.0	Tr	Tr	1 pint (576g)	18.4	4½
						½ pint 284ml (288g)	9.2	2¼
						500 ml bottle (507g)	16.2	4
						440ml can (446g)	14.3	3½
Vermouth, dry	3.0	¾	0.7	1.2	1.1	1 measure – 50 ml (50g)	1.5	½
Vermouth, sweet	15.9	4	3.7	6.1	6.1	1 measure – 50ml (52g)	8.3	2
Wine, mulled wine, homemade	20.2	5	13.1	3.5	3.5	small glass – 175 ml (175g)	35.4	8¾
						large glass – 250ml (251g)	50.7	12¾
Wine, red	0.2	0	Tr	0.1	0.1	small glass – 175 ml (175g)	0.4	0
						large glass – 250ml (251g)	0.5	¼
Wine, rose, medium	2.5	¾	0.0	1.7	0.8	small glass – 175 ml (176g)	4.4	1
						large glass – 250ml (251g)	6.3	1½
Wine, white, dry	0.6	¼	0.0	0.3	0.3	small glass – 175 ml (174g)	1.0	¼
						large glass – 250ml (249g)	1.5	½
Wine, white, medium	3.0	¾	N	1.4	1.2	small glass – 175 ml (176g)	5.3	1¼
						large glass – 250ml (251g)	7.5	2
Wine, white, sparkling	5.1	1¼	0.1	2.8	2.2	small glass – 175 ml (174g)	8.9	2¼
						large glass – 250ml (249g)	12.7	3¼
Wine, white, sweet	5.9	1½	0.1	3.3	2.6	small glass – 175 ml (178g)	10.5	2¾
						large glass – 250ml (254g)	15.0	3¾

Beans and pulses

Food name	Total sugars (g/100g)	Teaspoons (tsp) sugar/100g	Sucrose (g/100g)	Fructose (g/100g)	Glucose (g/100g)	Average portion size	Grams (g) sugar per average portion	Tsp sugar per average p
Baked beans, canned in barbecue sauce	4.8	1¼	2.8	1.1	0.9	1 large (390g) can	18.7	4¾
Baked beans, canned in tomato sauce	4.8	1¼	3.4	0.8	0.6	large (415g) can small (200g) can or snack pot small (150g) can	19.9 9.6 7.2	5 2½ 1¾
Baked beans, canned in tomato sauce, reduced sugar, reduced salt	3.3	0.8	1.9	0.8	0.6	large (415g) can small (200g) can	13.7 6.6	3½ 1¾
Baked beans, canned in tomato sauce, with pork sausages	4.0	1	2.8	0.7	0.5	large (415g) can small (200g) can	16.6 8.0	4¼ 2
Beans, aduki, whole, dried, boiled in water	0.5	¼	0.3	Tr	Tr	2 tablespoons (60g)	0.3	0
Beans, aduki, whole, dried, raw	1.0	¼	0.7	Tr	0.1	¼ 500g packet (125g)	1.3	¼
Beans, blackeye, whole, dried, boiled in water	1.1	¼	0.9	Tr	0.1	2 tablespoons (60g)	0.7	¼
Beans, blackeye, whole, dried, raw	2.9	¾	2.5	0.1	0.2	2 tablespoons (60g)	1.7	½
Beans, broad, dried, raw	5.9	1½	3.8	1.5	0.6	¼ 500g packet (125g)	7.4	1¾
Beans, butter, canned, re-heated, drained	1.1	¼	1.1	Tr	Tr	1 large (400g) can 1 small (215g) can	4.4 2.4	1 ½
Beans, butter, dried, boiled in water	1.5	½	1.5	Tr	Tr	2 tablespoons (60g)	0.9	¼
Beans, butter, dried, raw	3.6	1	3.6	Tr	Tr	¼ 500g packet (125g)	4.5	1¼
Beans, chick peas, canned, re-heated, drained	0.4	0	0.4	Tr	Tr	large (400g) can small (215g) can	1.6 0.9	½ ¼
Beans, chick peas, Kabuli, split, dried, boiled in water	1.0	¼	0.9	0.1	Tr	2 tablespoons (60g)	0.6	¼
Beans, chick peas, Kabuli, split, dried, raw	2.6	¾	2.4	0.2	Tr	¼ 500g packet (125g)	3.3	¾
Beans, chick peas, Kabuli, whole, dried, boiled in water	1.0	¼	0.9	0.1	Tr	2 tablespoons (60g)	0.6	¼
Beans, chick peas, Kabuli, whole, dried, raw	2.6	¾	2.4	0.2	Tr	¼ 500g packet (125g)	3.3	¾

Food name	Total sugars (g/100g)	Teaspoons (tsp) sugar/100g	Sucrose (g/100g)	Fructose (g/100g)	Glucose (g/100g)	Average portion size	Grams (g) sugar per average portion	Tsp sugar per average portion
Beans, chilli, canned, re-heated	2.9	¾	1.5	0.8	0.6	1 whole large (390g) can	11.3	2¾
Beans, haricot, whole, dried, boiled in water	0.8	¼	0.7	Tr	0.1	2 tablespoons (60g)	0.5	¼
Beans, haricot, whole, dried, raw	2.8	¾	2.5	0.1	0.2	¼ 500g packet (125g)	3.5	1
Beans, lilva, canned, drained	Tr	0	Tr	Tr	Tr	½ large 400g can (200g)	Tr	0
Beans, mung, dahl, dried, boiled in water	0.5	¼	0.3	0.1	0.1	1 heaped tablespoon (35g)	0.2	0
Beans, mung, dahl, dried, raw	1.5	½	1.0	0.3	0.2	¼ 500g packet (125g)	1.9	½
Beans, mung, whole, dried, boiled in water	0.5	¼	0.3	0.1	0.1	2 tablespoons (60g)	0.3	0
Beans, mung, whole, dried, raw	1.5	½	1.0	0.3	0.2	¼ 500g packet (125g)	1.9	½
Beans, pigeon peas, dahl, dried, boiled in water	0.6	¼	0.5	0.1	Tr	1 heaped tablespoon (35g)	0.2	0
Beans, pigeon peas, dahl, dried, raw	1.7	½	1.4	0.2	0.1	¼ 500g packet (125g)	2.1	½
Beans, pigeon peas, whole, dried, boiled in water	0.6	¼	0.5	0.1	Tr	2 tablespoons (60g)	0.4	0
Beans, pigeon peas, whole, dried, raw	1.7	½	1.4	0.2	0.1	¼ 500g packet (125g)	2.1	½
Beans, red kidney, canned in water, re-heated, drained	0.6	¼	0.5	Tr	0.1	large (410g) can / small (215g) can	2.5 / 1.3	¾ / ¼
Beans, red kidney, dried, boiled in water	1.0	¼	0.8	Tr	0.1	1 heaped tablespoon (35g)	0.4	0
Beans, red kidney, dried, raw	2.5	¾	2.2	0.1	0.2	¼ 500g packet (125g)	3.1	¾
Beans, soya, dried, boiled in water	2.1	½	1.9	0.2	0.1	2 tablespoons (60g)	1.3	¼
Beans, soya, dried, raw	5.5	1½	4.8	0.5	0.2	¼ 500g packet (125g)	6.9	1¾
Black gram, chilki urad dahl, dried, split, boiled in water	0.3	0	0.3	Tr	Tr	1 heaped tablespoon (35g)	0.1	0
Black gram, chilki urad dahl, split, dried, raw	1.3	¼	1.1	0.1	0.1	¼ 500g packet (125g)	1.6	½
Black gram, duhli urad dahl, split, dried, boiled in water	0.3	0	0.3	Tr	Tr	1 heaped tablespoon (35g)	0.1	0

Food name	Total sugars (g/100g)	Teaspoons (tsp) sugar/100g	Sucrose (g/100g)	Fructose (g/100g)	Glucose (g/100g)	Average portion size	Grams (g) sugar per average portion	Tsp sugar per average portion
Black gram, duhli urad dahl, split, dried, raw	1.3	¼	1.1	0.1	0.1	¼ 500g packet (125g)	1.6	½
Black gram, urad gram, whole, dried, boiled in water	0.3	0	0.3	Tr	Tr	1 heaped tablespoon (35g)	0.1	0
Black gram, urad gram, whole, dried, raw	1.3	¼	1.1	0.1	0.1	¼ 500g packet (125g)	1.6	½
Lentils, canned in tomato sauce, re-heated	0.7	¼	0.3	0.2	0.2	½ large 400g can (200g)	1.4	¼
Lentils, green and brown, whole, dried, boiled in water	0.4	0	0.4	Tr	Tr	1 heaped tablespoon (35g)	0.1	0
Lentils, green and brown, whole, dried, raw	1.2	¼	1.1	0.1	Tr	¼ 500g packet (125g)	1.5	½
Lentils, red, split, dried, boiled in water	0.8	¼	0.7	0.1	Tr	1 heaped tablespoon (35g)	0.3	0
Lentils, red, split, dried, raw	2.4	½	2.2	0.2	Tr	¼ 500g packet (125g)	3	¾
Peas, dried, boiled in unsalted water	2.4	½	2.2	0.1	0.1	2 tablespoons (60g)	1.4	¼
Peas, dried, raw	5.9	1½	5.9	Tr	Tr	¼ 500g packet (125g)	7.4	1¾
Peas, split, dried, boiled in water	0.9	¼	0.8	Tr	Tr	1 heaped tablespoon (35g)	0.3	0
Peas, split, dried, raw	1.9	½	1.7	0.1	0.1	¼ 500g packet (125g)	2.4	½
Re-fried beans	1.4	¼	0.8	0.2	0.3	large (435g) can / small (215g) can	6.1 / 3.0	1½ / ¾

Biscuits and crackers

Food name	Total sugars (g/100g)	Teaspoons (tsp) sugar/100g	Sucrose (g/100g)	Fructose (g/100g)	Glucose (g/100g)	Average portion size	Grams (g) sugar per average portion	Tsp sugar per average portion
Biscuits, cheese flavoured	2.7	¾	2.7	Tr	Tr	3g	0.1	0
Biscuits, cookies, chocolate chip, American style	40.5	10¼	40.5	Tr	Tr	50g	20.3	4
Biscuits, cookies, chocolate chip, standard	30.0	7½	30	Tr	Tr	9g	2.7	¾
Biscuits, digestive, half coated in chocolate	24.3	6	24.3	Tr	Tr	18g	4.4	1
Biscuits, digestive, plain	17.5	4	17.5	Tr	Tr	15g	2.6	¾
Biscuits, digestive, with oats, plain	25.9	6½	23.9	0.9	1.2	14g	3.6	1
Biscuits, fully coated with chocolate	39.3	10	33.3	Tr	Tr	24g	9.4	2¼
Biscuits, fully coated with chocolate, with cream	37.4	9¼	34.1	Tr	Tr	25g	9.4	2¼
Biscuits, fully coated with chocolate, with marshmallow	41.4	10¼	28.7	Tr	6	36g	14.9	3¾
Biscuits, ginger nuts	31.3	7¾	22.6	2.4	3	10g	3.1	¾
Biscuits, gingernut, homemade	32.6	8¼	16	8.2	8.2	10g	3.3	¾
Biscuits, iced	44.6	10½	44.6	Tr	Tr	12g	5.4	1¼
Biscuits, jam filled	33.0	8¼	19.4	2.1	6.1	17g	5.6	1½
Biscuits, oat based, chocolate, half coated	33.1	8¼	29.4	0.7	0.9	16g	5.3	1¼
Biscuits, plain, homemade	26.4	7½	26.2	Tr	Tr	10g	2.6	¾
Biscuits, plain, reduced fat	21.2	5¼	20.3	Tr	0.9	7g	1.5	½
Biscuits, sandwich, cream	29.9	7½	27.2	Tr	1.6	11g	3.3	¾
Biscuits, semi-sweet	20.3	5	19.7	Tr	0.6	7g	1.4	¼
Biscuits, short or sweet, half coated in chocolate	35.5	9	32.5	Tr	Tr	15g	5.3	1¼
Biscuits, short, sweet	23.8	6	22	0.6	0.6	13g (finger)	3.1	¾
Biscuits, wafer, filled	44.7	11¼	42.9	0.0	1.4	19g	8.5	2¼
Biscuits, wholemeal, homemade	4.2	1	0.9	Tr	Tr	10g	0.4	0
Brandy snaps, homemade	50.1	12½	37.3	6.3	6.3	15g	7.5	2
Crackers, wholemeal, homemade	0.8	¼	0.6	Tr	Tr	10g	0.1	0
Cream crackers	1.5	½	Tr	Tr	Tr	7g	0.1	0
Crispbread, rye	3.4	¾	2.8	Tr	Tr	10g	0.3	0

Food name	Total sugars (g/100g)	Teaspoons (tsp) sugar/100g	Sucrose (g/100g)	Fructose (g/100g)	Glucose (g/100g)	Average portion size	Grams (g) sugar per average portion	Tsp sugar per average portion
Fig Rolls	43.8	11	15.8	8.4	11.5	15g	6.6	1¾
Flapjacks, homemade	34.5	8¾	4.5	4.4	25.6	90g	31.1	7¾
Flapjacks, retail	29.2	7½	4.3	4.2	20.7	70g	20.4	5
Flapjacks, retail, chocolate covered	31.3	7¾	4.0	3.9	22.8	50g	15.7	4
Gingerbread, homemade	34.7	8¾	6.0	6.0	22.1	50g (man)	17.4	4¼
Jaffa cakes	51.6	13	8.5	1.8	35.1	13g	6.7	1¾
Macaroon, homemade	62.0	15½	Tr	Tr	62.0	28g	17.4	4¼
Matzos	4.2	1	0.0	0.0	0.0	5g	0.2	0
Oatcakes, homemade	0.3	0	Tr	Tr	0.3	17g	0.1	0
Oatcakes, plain, retail	3.2	¾	Tr	Tr	1.0	13g	0.4	0
Rice cakes, plain, low salt	0.9	¼	Tr	0.1	0.6	7g	0.1	0
Shortbread	15.6	4	Tr	Tr	15.6	20g	3.1	¾
Shortcake, caramel, chocolate covered, retail	36.2	9	1.8	2.0	27.8	14g	5.1	1¼

Bread, pastry, flour and baked goods

Food name	Total sugars (g/100g)	Teaspoons (tsp) sugar/100g	Sucrose (g/100g)	Fructose (g/100g)	Glucose (g/100g)	Average portion size	Grams (g) sugar per average portion	Tsp sugar per average portion
Bannocks, made with beremeal, homemade	3.1	¾	0.1	0.1	0.7	medium (150g) wedge	4.7	1¼
Bannocks, made with wheat flour, homemade	2.4	½	Tr	Tr	0.4	medium (150g) wedge	3.6	1
Bagels, plain	4.8	1¼	Tr	1.0	0.8	70g each	3.4	¾
Bread rolls, brown, crusty	1.9	½	N	N	N	48g each	0.9	¼
Bread rolls, brown, soft	2.8	¾	Tr	0.4	0.5	48g each	1.3	¼
Bread rolls, malted wheat	3.0	¾	Tr	0.6	0.3	56g each	1.7	½
Bread rolls, white, crusty	2.7	¾	Tr	0.2	Tr	50g each	1.4	¼
Bread rolls, white, soft	2.6	¾	Tr	0.2	0.2	45g each	1.1	¼
Bread rolls, wholemeal	2.6	¾	Tr	0.5	0.5	56g each	1.5	½
Bread, brown, average	3.4	¾	Tr	0.3	Tr	small loaf, 1 slice (25g)	0.9	¼
						large loaf, 1 medium slice (36g)	1.2	¼
						large loaf, 1 thick slice (44g)	1.5	½
Bread, brown, toasted	4.4	1¼	Tr	0.4	Tr	small loaf, 1 slice (23g)	1.0	¼
						large loaf, 1 medium slice (31g)	1.4	¼
						large loaf, 1 thick slice (40g)	1.8	½
Bread, ciabatta	3.1	¾	0.3	0.1	Tr	¼ whole 260g loaf (65g)	2	½
Bread, currant	14.4	3½	0.0	6.7	6.3	1 slice (50g)	7.2	1¾
Bread, currant, toasted	16.1	4	0.0	7.5	7.0	1 slice (48g)	7.7	2
Bread, focaccia, herb / garlic and coriander	2.6	¾	Tr	0.2	Tr	¼ whole 240g loaf (60g)	1.6	½
Bread, garlic and herb, retail	2.9	¾	Tr	0.2	0.1	1 slice (20g)	0.6	¼
Bread, hamburger buns	2.2	½	N	N	N	50g each	1.1	¼
Bread, malt, fruited	22.6	5¾	1.0	6.3	7.4	1 slice (35g)	7.9	2
Bread, malted wheat	2.9	¾	Tr	0.3	0.1	small loaf, 1 slice (25g)	0.7	¼
						large loaf, 1 medium slice (36g)	1.0	¼
						large loaf, 1 thick slice (44g)	1.3	¼
Bread, milk, white, sliced	4.5	1¼	Tr	0.3	0.3	1 slice (27g)	1.2	¼
Bread, naan, peshwari naan, takeaway and retail	1.6	½	1.6	Tr	Tr	155g	2.5	¾

Food name	Total sugars (g/100g)	Teaspoons (tsp) sugar/100g	Sucrose (g/100g)	Fructose (g/100g)	Glucose (g/100g)	Average portion size	Grams (g) sugar per average portion	Tsp sugar per average portion
Bread, naan, retail	3.1	¾	Tr	0.8	0.7	160g	5	1¼
Bread, pitta, white	3.0	¾	Tr	0.5	0.5	75g each mini, "picnic" (35g) each	1	¼
Bread, rye	1.8	½	N	N	N	1 slice (25g)	0.5	¼
Bread, seeded	3.8	1	N	N	N	small loaf, 1 average slice (30g)	1.1	¼
						large loaf, 1 medium slice (38g)	1.4	¼
						large loaf, 1 thick slice (55g)	2.1	½
Bread, soda, made with white flour, homemade	2.3	½	0.3	Tr	Tr	1 farl (130g)	3	¾
Bread, wheatgerm	3.8	1	Tr	0.6	0.2	small loaf, 1 slice (25g)	1.0	¼
						large loaf, 1 medium slice (36g)	1.4	¼
						large loaf, 1 thick slice (44g)	1.7	½
Bread, white, average	3.0	¾	Tr	0.2	Tr	small loaf, 1 slice (27g)	0.8	¼
						large loaf, 1 medium slice (35g)	1.0	¼
						large loaf, 1 thick slice (50g)	1.5	½
Bread, white, crusty bloomer, unsliced, fresh, large	2.8	¾	Tr	0.2	Tr	small loaf, 1 slice (27g)	0.8	¼
						large loaf, 1 medium slice (35g)	1.0	¼
						large loaf, 1 thick slice (50g)	1.4	¼
Bread, white, Danish style	3.0	¾	Tr	0.2	0.1	1 medium slice (20g)	0.6	¼
Bread, white, farmhouse or split tin	2.9	¾	Tr	0.2	Tr	1 slice (27g)	0.8	¼
Bread, white, French stick	2.8	¾	Tr	0.2	Tr	2" slice (40g)	1.1	¼
						6" slice (120g)	3.4	¾
Bread, white, premium	2.7	¾	Tr	0.2	Tr	small loaf, 1 slice (25g)	0.7	¼
						large loaf, 1 thin slice (31g)	0.8	¼
						large loaf, 1 medium slice (36g)	1.0	¼
						large loaf, 1 thick slice (44g)	1.2	¼
Bread, white, sliced	3.4	¾	Tr	0.2	Tr	small loaf, 1 slice (25g)	0.9	¼
						large loaf, 1 thin slice (31g)	1.1	¼
						large loaf, 1 medium slice (36g)	1.2	¼
						large loaf, 1 thick slice (44g)	1.5	½

Food name	Total sugars (g/100g)	Teaspoons (tsp) sugar/100g	Sucrose (g/100g)	Fructose (g/100g)	Glucose (g/100g)	Average portion size	Grams (g) sugar per average portion	Tsp sugar per average portion
Bread, white, sliced, fried	3.5	1	Tr	0.2	Tr	small loaf, 1 slice (35g)	1.2	¼
						large loaf, 1 thin slice (41g)	1.4	¼
						large loaf, 1 medium slice (46g)	1.6	½
						large loaf, 1 thick slice (54g)	1.9	½
Bread, white, toasted	4.1	1	Tr	0.2	Tr	small loaf, 1 slice (20g)	0.8	¼
						large loaf, 1 thin slice (22g)	0.9	¼
						large loaf, 1 medium slice (27g)	1.1	¼
						large loaf, 1 thick slice (34g)	1.4	¼
Bread, white, 'with added fibre'	3.5	1	Tr	0.3	0.1	small loaf, 1 slice (25g)	0.9	¼
						large loaf, 1 thin slice (31g)	1.1	¼
						large loaf, 1 medium slice (36g)	1.3	¼
						large loaf, 1 thick slice (44g)	1.5	½
Bread, white, 'with added fibre', toasted	4.2	1	Tr	0.4	0.1	small loaf, 1 slice (20g)	0.8	¼
						large loaf, 1 thin slice (22g)	0.9	¼
						large loaf, 1 medium slice (27g)	1.1	¼
						large loaf, 1 thick slice (34g)	1.4	¼
Bread, wholemeal, average	2.8	¾	Tr	0.4	0.2	small loaf, 1 slice (25g)	0.7	¼
						large loaf, 1 medium slice (36g)	1.0	¼
						large loaf, 1 thick slice (44g)	1.2	¼
Bread, wholemeal, toasted	3.2	¾	Tr	0.5	0.2	small loaf, 1 slice (23g)	0.7	¼
						large loaf, 1 medium slice (31g)	1.0	¼
						large loaf, 1 thick slice (40g)	1.3	¼
Breadsticks, plain	3.3	¾	Tr	Tr	Tr	7g each	0.2	0
Chapatis, made with fat, retail	1.8	½	N	N	N	60g each	1.1	¼
Chapatis, made without fat	1.6	½	N	N	N	55g each	0.9	¼
Cheese and onion rolls, pastry, retail	3.0	¾	0.4	0.3	0.4	70g each	2.1	½
Cheese straws/twists, retail	1.6	½	Tr	Tr	Tr	33g each	0.5	¼
Croissants	5.3	1¼	Tr	2.0	1.2	60g each	3.2	¾
Crumpets, toasted	3.1	¾	Tr	0.3	1.1	40g each	1.2	¼
Currant buns, retail	16.0	4	Tr	7.0	8.2	60g each	9.6	2 ½
Dumplings, homemade	0.2	0	0.1	0.0	0.0	70g each	0.1	0

Food name	Total sugars (g/100g)	Teaspoons (tsp) sugar/100g	Sucrose (g/100g)	Fructose (g/100g)	Glucose (g/100g)	Average portion size	Grams (g) sugar per average portion	Tsp sugar per average portion
Flour, chapati, brown	1.1	¼	0.9	Tr	Tr	1oz (28g)	0.3	0
Flour, chapati, white	0.6	¼	0.5	Tr	Tr	1oz (28g)	0.2	0
Flour, corn	Tr	0	Tr	0.0	Tr	1oz (28g)	Tr	0
Flour, gari (cassava flour)	Tr	0	Tr	Tr	Tr	1oz (28g)	Tr	0
Flour, gram	2.3	½	2.3	Tr	Tr	1oz (28g)	0.6	¼
Flour, rye	1.5	½	1.2	Tr	Tr	1oz (28g)	0.4	0
Flour, soya	6.4	1½	6.4	Tr	Tr	1oz (28g)	1.8	½
Flour, wheat, bread/strong, white	0.5	¼	0.4	Tr	Tr	1oz (28g)	0.1	0
Flour, wheat, brown	1.0	¼	0.9	Tr	Tr	1oz (28g)	0.3	0
Flour, wheat, brown, bread/strong	1.0	¼	0.6	Tr	Tr	1oz (28g)	0.3	0
Flour, wheat, white, plain, soft	0.6	¼	0.5	Tr	Tr	1oz (28g)	0.2	0
Flour, wheat, white, self raising	0.6	¼	0.5	Tr	Tr	1oz (28g)	0.2	0
Flour, wheat, wholemeal	1.4	¼	1.0	Tr	Tr	1oz (28g)	0.4	0
Flour, wheat, wholemeal, bread/strong	1.1	¼	0.8	Tr	Tr	1oz (28g)	0.3	0
Flour, wheat, wholemeal, self raising	1.1	¼	1.0	Tr	Tr	1oz (28g)	0.3	0
Milk bread, homemade	2.1	½	0.2	Tr	Tr	1 slice (27g)	0.6	¼
Minibreads, toasted, retail (e.g. Brioche)	3.3	¾	Tr	Tr	Tr	45g each	1.5	½
Mooli paratha, homemade	1.8	½	0.3	0.5	0.9	170g	3.1	¾
Muffins, bran, homemade	17.3	4¼	12.7	1.3	1.3	72g each	12.5	3¼
Muffins, English style, white	3.4	¾	Tr	0.8	0.5	68g each	2.3	½
Muffins, English style, white, toasted	3.8	1	Tr	0.8	0.5	64g each	2.4	½

Food name	Total sugars (g/100g)	Teaspoons (tsp) sugar/100g	Sucrose (g/100g)	Fructose (g/100g)	Glucose (g/100g)	Average portion size	Grams (g) sugar per average portion	Tsp sugar per average
Pancakes, savoury, made with semi-skimmed milk, homemade	3.8	1	0.1	Tr	Tr	68g each	2.6	¾
Pancakes, savoury, made with skimmed milk, homemade	3.9	1	0.1	Tr	Tr	68g each	2.7	¾
Pancakes, savoury, wholemeal, made with whole milk, homemade	4.0	1	0.3	Tr	Tr	68g each	2.7	¾
Papadums, takeaway	Tr	0	Tr	Tr	Tr	13g each	Tr	0
Paratha, homemade	0.7	¼	0.6	Tr	Tr	140g each	1.0	¼
Pastry, cheese, shortcrust, homemade	0.5	¼	0.2	Tr	Tr	1oz (28g)	0.1	0
Pastry, choux, cooked, homemade	0.2	0	0.2	Tr	Tr	1oz (28g)	0.1	0
Pastry, choux, uncooked, homemade	0.2	0	0.1	Tr	Tr	1oz (28g)	0.1	0
Pastry, filo, retail, cooked	3.1	¾	Tr	0.1	0.2	1 whole 45g sheet	1.4	¼
Pastry, filo, retail, uncooked	2.4	½	Tr	0.1	0.2	1 whole 45g sheet	1.1	¼
Pastry, flaky, cooked, homemade	0.6	¼	0.3	0.0	0.0	1oz (28g)	0.2	0
Pastry, flaky, uncooked, homemade	0.5	¼	0.2	0.0	0.0	1oz (28g)	0.1	0
Pastry, flaky/puff, retail, cooked	1.9	½	Tr	Tr	Tr	1 pastry square (62.4g)	1.2	¼
Pastry, flaky/puff, retail, uncooked	1.5	½	Tr	Tr	Tr	1 pastry square (62.4g)	0.9	¼
Pastry, shortcrust, cooked, homemade	0.6	¼	0.4	Tr	Tr	1oz (28g)	0.2	0
Pastry, shortcrust, retail, cooked	1.0	¼	Tr	Tr	0.4	1/6 500g block (83g)	0.8	¼
Pastry, shortcrust, retail, uncooked	0.9	¼	Tr	Tr	0.3	1/6 500g block (83g)	0.7	¼
Pastry, shortcrust, uncooked, homemade	0.5	¼	0.3	Tr	Tr	1oz (28g)	0.1	0
Pastry, wholemeal, cooked, homemade	1.2	¼	0.7	Tr	Tr	1oz (28g)	0.3	0

Food name	Total sugars (g/100g)	Teaspoons (tsp) sugar/100g	Sucrose (g/100g)	Fructose (g/100g)	Glucose (g/100g)	Average portion size	Grams (g) sugar per average portion	Tsp sugar per average portion
Pastry, wholemeal, uncooked, homemade	1.0	¼	0.6	Tr	Tr	1oz (28g)	0.3	0
Pizza base, raw	3.4	¾	Tr	0.3	0.3	small (100g) medium (200g) large (350–500g)	3.4 6.8 11.9– 17.0	¾ 1 ¾ 4– 4¼
Potato cakes, fried in oil	1.1	¼	0.3	0.2	0.2	65g each	0.7	¼
Puri, homemade	1.2	¼	0.5	Tr	Tr	70g	0.8	¼
Rusks	23.4	5¾	19.7	1.4	2.3	17g each	4	1
Scones, potato, homemade	1.4	¼	0.2	0.1	0.1	56g each	0.8	¼
Tortilla, wheat, soft	2.0	½	Tr	0.4	Tr	45g each	0.9	¼
Yorkshire pudding, made with semi-skimmed milk, homemade	3.5	1	0.1	Tr	Tr	80g each	2.8	¾
Yorkshire pudding, made with skimmed milk, homemade	3.6	1	0.1	Tr	Tr	80g each	2.9	¾
Yorkshire pudding, made with whole milk	3.4	¾	0.1	Tr	Tr	80g each	2.7	¾

Cakes and pastries

Food name	Total sugars (g/100g)	Teaspoons (tsp) sugar/100g	Sucrose (g/100g)	Fructose (g/100g)	Glucose (g/100g)	Average portion size	Grams (g) sugar per average portion	Tsp sugar per average portion
Banana bread, homemade	36.3	9	19.9	6.4	7.6	1 slice (85g)	30.1	7½
Brownies, chocolate, homemade	46.1	11½	45.9	0.0	0.0	60g each	27.7	7
Cake bars, chocolate	41.5	10½	33.3	1.0	2.1	30g each	12.5	3¼
Cake bars, not chocolate	41.9	10½	22.7	6.9	9.8	30g each	12.6	3¼
Cake mix	41.6	10½	39.1	Tr	0.1	1 whole (500g) pack	208	52
Cake rusks (South Asian sweet bread)	24.6	6¼	23.5	Tr	Tr	30g each	7.4	1¾
Cake, battenberg, retail	56.8	14¼	46.7	0.3	5.1	1 slice (32g)	18.2	4½
Cake, carrot, iced, retail	34.5	8¾	31.8	0.8	Tr	1 square (30g)	10.4	2½
Cake, carrot, with topping, homemade	23.7	6	20.8	1.2	1.3	1 slice (58g)	13.7	3½
Cake, cherry, homemade	40.0	10	20.7	4.2	7.9	1 slice (42g)	16.8	4¼
Cake, chocolate fudge	43.5	11	39.1	0.4	1.7	1 slice (98g)	42.6	10¾
Cake, chocolate, not filled, homemade	28.5	7¼	28.4	Tr	Tr	1 slice (48g)	13.7	3½
Cake, chocolate, with butter icing, homemade	35.7	9	35.5	Tr	Tr	1 slice (65g)	23.2	5¾
Cake, chocolate, with filling and icing, retail	36.6	9¼	33.2	Tr	1.4	40g	14.6	3¾
Cake, coconut, homemade	21.3	5¼	20.7	0.1	Tr	1 slice (40g)	8.5	2¼
Cake, fruit, retail	39.6	10	14.0	11.9	10.5	1 slice (60g)	23.8	6
Cake, fruit, rich, homemade	49.6	12½	13.7	15.4	17.3	1 slice (70g)	34.7	8¾
Cake, fruit, rich, iced, homemade	58.9	14¾	32.4	11.0	12.9	1 slice (70g)	41.2	10¼
Cake, fruit, wholemeal, homemade	29.2	7¼	17.2	5.3	5.6	1 slice (90g)	26.3	6½
Cake, lardy, homemade	10.0	2½	7.7	Tr	Tr	1 slice (55g)	5.5	1½
Cake, loaf, retail	33.5	8½	13.6	6.8	10.2	1 slice (30g)	10.1	2½
Cake, madeira, retail	36.5	9¼	35.5	0.5	0.5	1 slice (40g)	14.6	3¾
Cake, sponge, fatless, homemade	30.6	7¾	30.6	Tr	Tr	1 slice (38g)	11.6	3
Cake, sponge, homemade	30.3	7½	30.1	Tr	Tr	1 slice (38g)	11.5	3
Cake, sponge, jam filled, retail	47.7	12	35.7	3.9	8.1	1 slice (60g)	28.6	7¼
Cake, sponge, soft iced, retail	39.0	9¾	35.5	Tr	Tr	1 small individual (28g)	10.9	2¾

Food name	Total sugars (g/100g)	Teaspoons (tsp) sugar/100g	Sucrose (g/100g)	Fructose (g/100g)	Glucose (g/100g)	Average portion size	Grams (g) sugar per average portion	Tsp sugar per average portion
Cake, sponge, with butter icing, homemade	40.0	10	39.8	Tr	Tr	1 slice (60g)	24	6
Cake, sponge, with dairy cream and jam, frozen	24.3	6	18.1	0.7	3.0	1 slice (39g)	9.4	2¼
Cake, sponge, with jam and butter cream, retail	37.6	9½	28.2	1.0	3.5	1 slice (100g)	37.6	9½
Cake, Swiss roll, homemade	42.2	10½	30.0	3.6	6.6	1 slice (28g)	11.8	3
Cake, Swiss rolls, chocolate covered and filled, retail	41.2	10¼	33.8	Tr	4.1	25g each	10.3	2½
Cakes from 'healthy eating' ranges	47.4	11¾	41.9	1.7	2.8	30g each	14.2	3½
Cakes, crispie, homemade	43.0	10¾	42.2	0.4	0.4	25g each	10.8	2¾
Cakes, fancy iced, individual, retail	44.1	11	40.5	Tr	1.5	39g each	17.2	4¼
Cheesecake, fruit, frozen	25.0	6¼	19.4	1.6	1.8	90g	22.5	5¾
Cheesecake, fruit, individual	25.4	6¼	18.1	2.0	2.3	90g	22.9	5¾
Cheesecake, fruit, low fat, individual	20.2	5	13.1	1.2	5.1	90g	18.2	4½
Cheesecake, homemade	15.5	4	13.8	0.1	0.0	1 slice (120g)	18.6	4¾
Cheesecake, not fruit, frozen	19.4	4¾	15.4	0.4	0.4	1 slice (120g)	23.3	5¾
Chelsea buns, homemade	21.0	5¼	4.4	4.3	11.2	78g	16.4	4
Choux buns, homemade	0.9	¼	Tr	Tr	0.1	112g each	1	¼
Corn pudding, homemade (West Indian dish)	5.9	1½	3.4	0.2	0.3	100g	5.9	1½
Doughnuts, custard-filled	15.3	3¾	9.6	2.2	1.9	75g each	11.5	3
Doughnuts, ring, iced	16.2	4	1.7	0.8	13.7	75g each	12.2	3
Doughnuts, with jam	20.3	5	11.4	5.5	Tr	75g each	15.2	3¾
Eccles cakes, retail	34.0	8½	10.8	15.4	3.3	45g each	15.3	3¾
Flan case, pastry, homemade	11.9	3	Tr	Tr	11.8	large case (200g)	23.8	6
Flan case, sponge, homemade	34.6	8¾	Tr	Tr	34.6	small case (96g) large case (200g)	33.2 69.2	8 ¼ 17¼
Flan, pastry, with fruit, homemade	11.2	2¾	3.6	4.1	3.6	95g	10.6	2¾
Flan, sponge, with fruit, homemade	15.8	4	9.2	3.5	3.1	95g	15	3¾

Food name	Total sugars (g/100g)	Teaspoons (tsp) sugar/100g	Sucrose (g/100g)	Fructose (g/100g)	Glucose (g/100g)	Average portion size	Grams (g) sugar per average portion	Tsp sugar per average portion
Gateau, chocolate based, frozen	17.4	3¾	11.5	1.8	2.4	1 portion (90g)	15.7	4
Gateau, fruit, frozen	14.9	3¾	10.1	1.5	2.0	1 slice (85g)	12.7	3¼
Hot cross buns, homemade	23.4	5¾	5.0	4.1	11.7	50g each	11.7	3
Iced buns, retail	25.8	6½	6.4	7.0	11.4	65g each	16.8	4¼
Jam tarts, retail	32.1	8	10.9	3.7	9.4	34g each	10.9	2¾
Macaroon, homemade	62.0	15½	62.0	Tr	Tr	28g each	17.4	4¼
Mince pies, homemade, individual	29.0	7¼	0.3	14.1	14.3	55g each	16	4
Mince pies, retail	35.5	9	3.4	11.9	16.6	55g each	19.5	5
Muffins, American style, chocolate chip, homemade	28.2	7	Tr	Tr	27.0	85g each	24	6
Muffins, American, chocolate, retail	30.9	7¾	0.6	0.1	28.3	85g each	26.3	6½
Muffins, American, not chocolate, retail	27.7	7	1.0	0.7	24.3	85g each	23.5	6
Pastries, Asian	22.6	5¾	N	N	N	95g each	21.5	5½
Pastries, chocolate eclairs, cream filled, retail	24.0	6	18.4	Tr	2.7	90g each	21.6	5½
Pastries, chocolate eclairs, fresh, homemade	26.0	6½	25.5	Tr	Tr	90g each	23.4	5¾
Pastries, cream filled, retail	27.3	6¾	20.8	1.0	2.7	60g each	16.4	4
Pastries, Danish, retail	17.3	4¼	9.6	2.7	3.3	medium (110g)	19	4¾
Pastries, Greek, baklava, retail	29.0	7¼	9.0	8.6	9.7	100g	29	7¼
Rock cakes, homemade	32.0	8	6.2	6.0	19.2	45g each	14.4	3½
Scones, cheese, homemade	1.9	½	Tr	Tr	0.3	48g each	0.9	¼
Scones, fruit, retail	18.9	4¾	3.0	2.7	9.9	48g each	9.1	2¼
Scones, fruit, wholemeal, homemade	13.9	3½	4.5	4.5	3.2	50g each	7	1¾
Scones, plain, homemade	5.4	1¼	Tr	Tr	3.5	48g each	2.6	¾
Scones, plain, retail	12.7	3¼	0.9	Tr	10.4	48g each	6.1	1½
Scones, wholemeal, homemade	5.6	1½	Tr	Tr	3.6	50g each	2.8	¾
Scotch pancakes, homemade	7.7	2	Tr	Tr	5.7	30g each	2.3	½
Scotch pancakes, retail	21.5	5½	2.0	1.6	14.1	45g each	9.7	2½
Strudel, fruit filled, retail, frozen	10.6	2¾	2.6	4.3	3.2	1 slice (115g)	12.2	3
Tart, bakewell, homemade	22.7	5¾	16.0	1.9	3.6	1 slice (120g)	27.2	6¾

Food name	Total sugars (g/100g)	Teaspoons (tsp) sugar/100g	Sucrose (g/100g)	Fructose (g/100g)	Glucose (g/100g)	Average portion size	Grams (g) sugar per average portion	Tsp sugar per average portion
Tart, custard, large, homemade	5.9	1½	3.1	Tr	0.1	95g	5.6	1½
Tart, mincemeat, one crust, homemade	37.6	9½	0.4	18.4	18.5	95g	35.7	9
Tartlets, strawberry, homemade	7.7	2	5.6	1.0	1.0	individual (21g) each	1.6	½
						'party' size (6g) each	0.5	¼
Tarts, bakewell, iced, retail	45.2	11¼	35.5	1.1	3.5	46g	20.8	5¼
Tarts, custard, individual	14.2	3½	11.2	Tr	0.9	1 individual tart (94g)	13.3	3¼
						1 slice of large tart (140g)	19.9	5
Tarts, jam, homemade	37.4	9¼	10.0	8.0	14.8	35g each	13.1	3¼
Tarts, jam, wholemeal, homemade	37.4	9¼	10.3	8.0	14.7	35g each	13.1	3¼
Torte, fruit	17.4	4¼	13.0	0.6	1.3	1 slice (90g)	15.7	4
Welsh cakes, homemade	31.5	8	20.8	4.9	5.1	28g each	8.8	2¼
Welsh cheesecakes, homemade	22.5	5¾	15.7	1.9	3.6	28g each	6.3	1½

Cooked dishes containing meat and poultry

Food name	Total sugars (g/100g)	Teaspoons (tsp) sugar/100g	Sucrose (g/100g)	Fructose (g/100g)	Glucose (g/100g)	Average portion size	Grams (g) sugar per average portion	Tsp sugar per average portion
Beef bourguignon, homemade	0.9	¼	0.2	0.3	0.3	210g	1.9	½
Beef bourguignonne, made with lean beef, homemade	0.8	¼	0.2	0.2	0.3	210g	1.7	½
Beef olives, homemade	0.3	0	0.1	0.1	0.1	1 thick slice (45g)	0.1	0
Beef steak pudding, homemade	0.8	¼	0.3	0.2	0.3	230g	1.8	½
Beef Stroganoff, homemade	2.1	½	0.4	0.4	0.5	210g	4.4	1
Beef Wellington, homemade	0.7	¼	0.0	0.0	0.1	200g	1.4	¼
Beef, mince patties, barbecued	0.0	0	0.0	0.0	0.0	95g each	0	0
Beef, mince, stewed	0.0	0	0.0	0.0	0.0	small portion (100g)	0.0	0
						medium portion (140g)	0.0	0
						large portion (220g)	0.0	0
Beef, mince, with vegetables, stewed	2.3	½	0.9	0.6	0.8	270g	6.2	1½
Beef, minced, stewed with onions	0.6	¼	0.2	0.2	0.2	small portion (100g)	0.6	¼
						medium portion (140g)	0.8	¼
						large portion (220g)	1.3	¼
Beef, stir-fried with green peppers, homemade	3.8	1	2.1	0.9	0.8	360g	13.7	3½
Bolognese sauce (with meat), homemade	2.6	¾	0.4	1.1	1.1	240g	6.2	1½
Burger, beef, with bun, fried or grilled, homemade	1.1	¼	N	N	N	quarterpounder (180g)	2	½
Burger, chicken/turkey, coated, retail, grilled	0.9	¼	0.2	Tr	0.2	90g	0.8	¼
Cabbage leaves, stuffed with lamb and rice, homemade	1.6	½	0.3	0.6	0.7	8g each	0.3	0
Carbonnade of Beef, homemade	2.7	¾	0.9	0.5	0.6	small portion (180g)	4.9	1¼
						medium portion (260g)	7.0	1¾
						large portion (360g)	9.7	1½

Food name	Total sugars (g/100g)	Teaspoons (tsp) sugar/100g	Sucrose (g/100g)	Fructose (g/100g)	Glucose (g/100g)	Average portion size	Grams (g) sugar per average portion	Tsp sugar per average portion
Casserole, beef, made with cook-in sauce	2.7	¾	0.9	0.9	0.8	small portion (180g)	4.9	1¼
						medium portion (260g)	7.0	1¾
						large portion (360g)	9.8	1½
Casserole, pork and apple, homemade	4.3	1	1.0	2.2	1.0	small portion (180g)	7.7	2
						medium portion (260g)	11.2	2¾
						large portion (360g)	15.5	4
Casserole, pork, made with cook-in sauce	2.3	½	0.7	0.8	0.7	small portion (180g)	4.1	1
						medium portion (260g)	6.0	1½
						large portion (360g)	8.3	2
Casserole, rabbit, homemade	1.1	¼	0.5	0.3	0.3	small portion (180g)	2.0	½
						medium portion (260g)	2.9	¾
						large portion (360g)	4.0	1
Casserole, sausage, homemade	2.0	½	0.9	0.3	0.6	small portion (180g)	3.6	1
						medium portion (260g)	5.2	1¼
						large portion (360g)	7.2	1¾
Chicken chasseur, homemade	1.1	¼	0.5	0.3	0.3	small portion (180g)	2.0	½
						medium portion (260g)	2.9	¾
						large portion (360g)	4.0	1
Chicken fricassee, homemade	1.5	½	0.3	0.5	0.5	small portion (180g)	2.7	¾
						medium portion (260g)	3.9	1
						large portion (360g)	5.4	1¼

Food name	Total sugars (g/100g)	Teaspoons (tsp) sugar/100g	Sucrose (g/100g)	Fructose (g/100g)	Glucose (g/100g)	Average portion size	Grams (g) sugar per average portion	Tsp sugar per average portion
Chicken fricassee, reduced fat, homemade	2.0	½	0.3	0.5	0.5	small portion (180g)	3.6	1
						medium portion (260g)	5.2	1¼
						large portion (360g)	7.2	1¾
Chicken in white sauce, canned	0.0	0	0.0	0.0	0.0	small (200g) can	0.0	0
						large (400g) can	0.0	0
Chicken in white sauce, made with semi-skimmed milk	2.3	½	0.0	Tr	Tr	small portion (180g)	4.1	1
						medium portion (260g)	6.0	1½
						large portion (360g)	8.3	2
Chicken in white sauce, made with whole milk	2.2	½	0.0	Tr	Tr	small portion (180g)	4.0	1
						medium portion (260g)	5.7	1½
						large portion (360g)	7.9	2
Chicken, stir-fried with mushrooms and cashew nuts, homemade	2.2	½	0.8	0.6	0.7	400g	8.8	2¼
Chicken, stir-fried with peppers in black bean sauce, homemade	2.4	½	1.0	0.7	0.6	400g	9.6	2½
Chicken, stir-fried with rice and vegetables, retail, reheated	3.9	1	1.0	1.1	1.8	400g	15.6	4
Chilli con carne, homemade	2.9	¾	0.6	1.1	1.1	220g (no rice)	6.4	1½
Chilli con carne, retail, reheated, with rice	1.6	½	N	N	N	ready meal for one (290g)	4.6	1¼
Chow mein, beef, retail, reheated	2.4	½	1.2	0.0	N	350g	8.4	2
Chow mein, pork and chicken, homemade	1.5	½	N	N	N	350g	5.3	1¼
Coq au vin, homemade	0.4	0	0.1	0.1	0.1	small portion (180g)	0.7	¼
						medium portion (260g)	1.0	¼
						large portion (360g)	1.4	¼

Food name	Total sugars (g/100g)	Teaspoons (tsp) sugar/100g	Sucrose (g/100g)	Fructose (g/100g)	Glucose (g/100g)	Average portion size	Grams (g) sugar per average portion	Tsp sugar per average portion
Coq au vin, homemade, weighed with bone	0.3	0	0.1	0.1	0.1	small portion (180g)	0.5	¼
						medium portion (260g)	0.8	¼
						large portion (360g)	1.9	½
Corned beef hash, homemade	1.9	½	0.8	0.5	0.6	198g	3.8	1
Curry, beef and spinach, homemade	2.8	¾	0.4	1.1	1.2	350g	9.8	2½
Curry, beef, homemade	0.6	¼	0.2	0.2	0.2	350g	2.1	½
Curry, beef, reduced fat, homemade	0.7	¼	0.2	0.2	0.3	350g	2.5	¾
Curry, beef, retail, reheated	4.5	1¼	0.7	1.6	1.5	200g	9	2¼
Curry, beef, retail, reheated, with rice	2.6	¾	0.4	0.9	0.9	400g	10.4	2½
Curry, chicken balti, retail	3.5	1	N	N	N	200g	7	1¾
Curry, chicken korma, homemade	2.8	¾	0.4	0.3	0.4	350g	9.8	2½
Curry, chicken tandoori, retail, reheated	1.0	¼	0.1	0.2	0.3	200g	2	½
Curry, chicken tikka masala, retail, reheated	3.6	1	0.8	0.9	0.7	200g	7.2	1¾
Curry, chicken vindaloo, homemade	1.7	½	1.0	0.3	0.4	350g	6	1½
Curry, chicken vindaloo, reduced fat, homemade	1.8	½	1.0	0.3	0.4	350g	6.3	1½
Curry, chicken, average, retail, reheated	4.4	1	0.7	1.6	1.5	200g	8.8	2¼
Curry, chicken, average, retail, reheated with rice	2.4	½	0.4	0.9	0.8	400g	9.6	2½
Curry, chicken, made with cook-in sauce	3.9	1	1.3	1.4	1.2	350g	13.7	3½
Curry, lamb biryani, homemade	2.0	½	0.2	0.5	0.6	350g	7	1¾
Curry, lamb biryani, reduced fat, homemade	2.0	½	0.2	0.5	0.6	350g	7	1¾
Curry, lamb rogan josh, homemade	3.0	¾	0.6	1.1	1.2	350g	10.5	2¾
Curry, lamb vindaloo, homemade	1.8	½	1.0	0.3	1.4	350g	6.3	1½

Food name	Total sugars (g/100g)	Teaspoons (tsp) sugar/100g	Sucrose (g/100g)	Fructose (g/100g)	Glucose (g/100g)	Average portion size	Grams (g) sugar per average portion	Tsp sugar per average p
Curry, lamb, made with cook-in sauce	3.9	1	1.3	1.4	1.2	350g	13.7	3½
Devilled kidneys, homemade	1.5	½	0.2	0.4	0.3	1 tablespoon (40g)	0.6	¼
Duck a l'orange, including fat and skin, homemade	0.9	¼	0.3	0.3	0.3	185g	1.7	½
Duck with pineapple, homemade	4.9	1¼	2.7	1.0	1.1	185g	9.1	2¼
Duck, crispy, chinese style	0.0	0	0.0	0.0	0.0	125g	0	0
Enchiladas, beef, homemade	2.7	¾	0.5	1.0	0.9	180g each	4.9	1¼
Faggots in gravy, retail, reheated	1.7	½	0.3	0.3	0.5	2 faggots (150g)	2.6	¾
Frankfurter with bun	2.1	½	Tr	0.1	0.2	small (32g) large (85g) each	0.7 1.8	¼ ½
Frankfurter with bun, ketchup, fried onions and mustard	6.7	1¾	2.4	1.5	1.8	small (62g) large (120g) each	4.2 8.0	1 2
Goulash, homemade	1.7	½	0.4	0.6	0.7	210g	3.6	1
Hot pot, lamb/beef with potatoes, retail, reheated	1.0	¼	0.4	0.3	0.3	400g	4	1
Irish stew, canned	1.2	¼	0.4	0.0	0.4	large can (400g)	4.8	1¼
Kebabs, pork and pineapple, homemade	6.1	1½	1.0	2.6	2.2	90g	5.5	1½
Kheema, beef, homemade	2.6	¾	1.3	0.6	0.7	350g	9.1	2¼
Kheema, lamb, homemade	2.4	½	1.3	0.6	0.6	350g	8.4	2
Kheema, lamb, reduced fat, homemade	1.6	½	0.6	0.5	0.5	350g	5.6	1½
Lamb stir-fried with vegetables, homemade	2.0	½	0.8	0.6	0.6	400g	8	2
Lamb's heart casserole, homemade	0.6	¼	N	N	N	210g	1.3	¼
Lancashire hotpot, homemade	1.4	¼	0.5	0.4	0.5	210g	2.9	¾
Lemon chicken, homemade	3.3	¾	3.2	0.1	Tr	small portion (180g) medium portion (260g) large portion (360g)	5.9 8.6 11.9	1½ 2¼ 3
Liver and onions, stewed, homemade	4.3	1	1.5	1.2	1.6	142g	6.1	1½

Food name	Total sugars (g/100g)	Teaspoons (tsp) sugar/100g	Sucrose (g/100g)	Fructose (g/100g)	Glucose (g/100g)	Average portion size	Grams (g) sugar per average portion	Tsp sugar per average portion
Meat buns, Chinese	9.0	2¼	N	N	N	1 small bun (60g)	5.4	1¼
						1 large bun (112g)	10.1	2½
Meat loaf, homemade	1.5	½	N	N	N	1 thin slice (160g)	2.4	½
Meatballs, pork and beef, in tomato sauce, homemade	2.8	¾	0.1	1.4	1.1	6 meatballs (80g)	1.2	¼
Moussaka, homemade	2.7	¾	0.2	0.7	0.9	400g	10.8	2¾
Moussaka, retail, reheated	2.0	½	0.0	0.6	0.4	325g	6.5	1¾
Pastichio (Greek dish)	2.8	¾	0.3	0.6	0.6	400g	11.2	2¾
Peppers, stuffed with beef, rice and vegetables, homemade	2.5	¾	0.2	1.1	1.0	1 pepper (350g)	8.8	2¼
Pie, beef, puff or shortcrust pastry, family size, retail	1.2	¼	0.4	0.2	0.2	1 slice (150g)	1.8	½
Pie, beef, puff or shortcrust pastry, individual, retail	1.2	¼	0.2	0.1	0.2	140g	1.7	½
Pie, chicken and mushroom, single crust, homemade	2.0	½	0.0	0.1	0.1	1 slice (150g)	3	¾
Pie, chicken, individual, baked	1.6	½	0.2	0.1	0.1	140g	2.2	½
Pie, Cottage, homemade	1.6	½	N	N	N	310g	5	1¼
Pie, Cottage/Shepherd's, reheated	1.6	½	0.3	0.2	0.3	310g	5	1¼
Pie, fish, white fish, homemade	1.5	½	0.1	0.2	0.2	250g	3.8	1
Pie, fish, white fish, retail, baked	1.8	½	0.3	Tr	0.2	320g	5.8	1½
Pie, game, homemade	3.4	¾	1.0	1.1	1.2	1 slice (175g)	6	1½
Pie, steak and kidney, double crust, homemade	0.9	¼	0.0	Tr	Tr	1 slice (150g)	1.4	¼
Pie, steak and kidney, single crust, homemade	0.6	¼	0.0	Tr	Tr	1 slice (150g)	0.9	¼
Pie, turkey, single crust, homemade	2.4	½	0.4	0.1	0.1	1 slice (150g)	3.6	1
Pork, stir-fried with vegetables, homemade	1.2	¼	0.4	0.4	0.4	400g	4.8	1¼
Pork, sweet and sour, homemade	7.8	2	5.5	1.1	1.2	300g	23.4	5¾
Pork, sweet and sour, made with sweet and sour cook in sauce	10.0	2½	5.0	2.5	2.5	300g	30	7½

Food name	Total sugars (g/100g)	Teaspoons (tsp) sugar/100g	Sucrose (g/100g)	Fructose (g/100g)	Glucose (g/100g)	Average portion size	Grams (g) sugar per average portion	Tsp sugar per average portion
Salmis of pheasant, homemade	1.4	¼	0.6	0.4	0.4	160g	2.2	½
Shepherd's pie, homemade	0.9	¼	0.2	0.2	0.2	310g	2.8	¾
Shish kebab in pitta bread with salad	1.3	¼	Tr	0.4	0.4	230g	3.0	¾
Shish kebab, meat only	0.0	0	0.0	0.0	0.0	85g	0.0	0
Shish kebabs, with onions and peppers, homemade	3.0	¾	0.6	1.2	1.2	140g	4.2	1
Steak and kidney pudding, homemade	0.8	¼	0.3	0.2	0.3	small (230g)	1.8	½
						large (450g)	3.6	1
Stew, beef, homemade	2.0	½	1.1	0.4	0.5	medium portion (270g)	5.4	1¼
						large portion (340g)	6.8	1¾
Stew, beef, with dumplings, homemade	1.6	½	0.9	0.3	0.4	medium portion + 1 dumpling (340g)	5.4	1¼
						large portion + 1 dumpling (410g)	6.7	1¾
						large portion + 2 dumplings (480g)	7.7	2
Stew, Irish, homemade	1.9	½	0.9	0.5	0.6	medium portion (270g)	5.1	1¼
						large portion (340g)	6.5	1¾
Stew, Irish, made with lean lamb, homemade	1.8	½	0.7	0.5	0.6	medium portion (270g)	4.9	1¼
						large portion (340g)	6.1	1½
Stewed steak with gravy, canned	Tr	Tr	Tr	Tr	Tr	large can (400g)	Tr	0
Toad in the hole, homemade	3.3	¾	0.1	Tr	0.7	310g	10.2	2½
Toad in the hole, made with skimmed milk and reduced fat sausages, homemade	3.8	1	0.1	Tr	0.8	310g	11.8	3
Turkey, stir-fried with vegetables, homemade	2.1	½	0.1	1.1	0.9	400g	8.4	2
Venison in red wine and port, homemade	1.6	½	0.5	0.4	0.5	260g	4.2	1

Cooking and baking ingredients, syrups and jams

Food name	Total sugars (g/100g)	Teaspoons (tsp) sugar/100g	Sucrose (g/100g)	Fructose (g/100g)	Glucose (g/100g)	Average portion size	Grams (g) sugar per average portion	Tsp sugar per average portion
Agar, dried	Tr	0	0.0	0.0	0.0	25g pack	Tr	0
Almonds, flaked and ground	4.2	1	4.2	Tr	Tr	1 tablespoon (12g)	0.5	¼
Arrowroot	Tr	0	Tr	0.0	Tr	1 heaped tablespoon (30g)	Tr	0
Baking powder	0.0	0	0.0	0.0	0.0	1 level teaspoon (4g)	0	0
Beef extract	0.4	0	Tr	0.2	0.2	1 heaped teaspoon (18g)	0.3	0
						1 level teaspoon (9g)	0.0	0
Bicarbonate of soda	0.0	0	0.0	0.0	0.0	1 level teaspoon (4g)	0	0
Breadcrumbs, retail	5.0	1¼	0.3	0.5	0.2	1 tablespoon (15g)	0.8	¼
Build up, powder, shake, assorted flavours	62.0	15½	N	N	N	30g sachet	18.6	4¾
Build-up powder, soup, assorted flavours	14.3	3½	N	N	N	30g sachet	4.3	1
Carob powder	31.3	7¾	23.3	3.7	4.3	1 heaped teaspoon (6g)	1.9	½
						1 level teaspoon (2g)	0.6	¼
Cocoa butter	0.0	0	0.0	0.0	0.0	1 teaspoon (5g)	0	0
Coconut, desiccated	6.4	1½	5.6	0.8	Tr	¼ 250g pack (62.5g)	4	1
Coconut cream	5.9	1½	5.8	0.1	Tr	1 whole 250ml carton (270g)	15.9	4
Coconut, creamed block	7.0	1¾	6.9	0.1	Tr	¼ 200g block (50g)	3.5	1
Cocoa powder	Tr	0	0.0	0.0	0.0	1 heaped teaspoon (6g)	Tr	0
						1 level teaspoon (2g)	Tr	0
Coconut milk	4.9	1¼	4.6	Tr	0.3	1 large can (400g)	19.6	5
Coconut milk, reduced fat, retail	1.1	0.3	N	N	N	1 large can (400g)	4.4	1
Coconut milk, retail	2.0	0.5	N	N	N	1 large can (400g)	8	2

Food name	Total sugars (g/100g)	Teaspoons (tsp) sugar/100g	Sucrose (g/100g)	Fructose (g/100g)	Glucose (g/100g)	Average portion size	Grams (g) sugar per average portion	Tsp sugar per average portion
Complan powder, original and sweet	42.8	10¾	4.9	0.0	0.4	55g sachet	23.5	6
Complan powder, savoury	6.2	1½	0.2	0.1	1.6	55g sachet	3.4	¾
Complan powder, savoury, made up with water	1.4	¼	0.0	0.0	0.4	255g	3.6	1
Complan powder, sweet, made up with semi-skimmed milk	13.0	3¼	1.1	0.0	0.1	262g	34.1	8½
Complan powder, sweet, made up with skimmed milk	13.1	3¼	1.1	0.0	0.1	262g	34.3	8½
Complan powder, sweet, made up with water	9.6	2½	1.1	0.0	0.1	255g	24.5	6¼
Complan powder, sweet, made up with whole milk	12.9	3¼	1.1	0.0	0.1	261g	33.7	8½
Cream of tartar	0.0	0	0.0	0.0	0.0	1 level teaspoon (4g)	0	0
Custard, confectioners'	19.0	4¾	15.3	Tr	Tr	110g	83.6	21
Fruit spread	30.7	7¾	0.4	16.7	13.6	1 heaped teaspoon (18g)	5.5	1½
						1 level teaspoon (8g)	2.5	¾
Gelatine	0.0	0	0.0	0.0	0.0	1 13g leaf	0	0
Glucose liquid	40.2	10	0.0	0.0	N	1 heaped teaspoon (17g)	6.8	1¾
						1 level teaspoon (8g)	3.2	¾
Honey	76.4	19	Tr	41.8	34.6	1 heaped teaspoon (17g)	13.0	3¼
						1 level teaspoon (8g)	6.1	1½
						average spreading on 1 slice bread (20g)	15.3	3¾
Icing, butter, homemade	62.8	15¾	62.3	0.1	0.1	50g	31.4	7¾
Icing, fondant, homemade	88.9	22¼	87.8	Tr	Tr	30g	26.7	6¾
Icing, glace, homemade	88.0	22	88.0	0.0	0.0	30g	26.4	6½
Icing, Royal, homemade	92.4	23	92.4	Tr	Tr	65g	60.1	15
Jaggery	89.3	22¼	N	N	N	1 level teaspoon (4g)	3.6	1

Food name	Total sugars (g/100g)	Teaspoons (tsp) sugar/100g	Sucrose (g/100g)	Fructose (g/100g)	Glucose (g/100g)	Average portion size	Grams (g) sugar per average portion	Tsp sugar per average portion
Jam, fruit with edible seeds	69.0	17¼	18.7	14.9	27.4	1 heaped teaspoon (18g)	12.4	3
						1 level teaspoon (8g)	5.5	1½
Jam, no added sugar	7.0	1¾	0.2	3.9	2.9	1 heaped teaspoon (18g)	1.3	¼
						1 level teaspoon (8g)	0.6	¼
Jam, reduced sugar	31.9	8	6.5	15.0	10.4	1 heaped teaspoon (18g)	5.7	1½
						1 level teaspoon (8g)	2.6	¾
Jam, stone fruit	69.3	17¼	18.8	14.9	27.5	1 heaped teaspoon (18g)	12.5	3¼
						1 level teaspoon (8g)	5.5	1½
Lemon curd	52.5	13¼	15.6	9.9	21.4	1 heaped teaspoon (18g)	9.5	2½
						1 level teaspoon (8g)	4.2	1
Lemon curd, homemade	50.7	12¾	50.3	0.2	0.1	1 heaped teaspoon (18g)	9.1	2¼
						1 level teaspoon (8g)	4.1	1
Marmalade	69.5	17½	18.8	15.0	27.6	1 heaped teaspoon (18g)	12.5	3¼
						1 level teaspoon (8g)	5.6	1½
Mincemeat	62.1	15½	0.6	30.8	30.7	1/8 411g jar (50g)	31.1	7¾
Mincemeat, vegetarian, homemade	42.5	10¾	15.8	10.8	12.5	1/8 411g jar (50g)	21.3	5¼
Molasses	59.4	14¾	35.1	12.9	11.5	1 heaped teaspoon (18g)	10.7	2¾
						1 level teaspoon (9g)	5.3	1¼
Peanut butter, smooth	6.7	1¾	6.7	0.0	0.0	thickly spread on one slice (20g)	1.3	¼
						thinly spread on one slice (12g)	0.8	¼
Peanut butter, wholegrain	4.4	1	4.4	0.0	0.0	thickly spread on one slice (20g)	0.9	¼
						thinly spread on one slice (12g)	0.5	¼

Food name	Total sugars (g/100g)	Teaspoons (tsp) sugar/100g	Sucrose (g/100g)	Fructose (g/100g)	Glucose (g/100g)	Average portion size	Grams (g) sugar per average portion	Tsp sugar per average portion
Peel, mixed	51.2	12 ¾	8.1	3.8	16.7	25g	12.8	3¼
Redcurrant jelly	63.8	16	21.0	21.4	21.4	1 heaped teaspoon (18g)	11.5	3
						1 level teaspoon (8g)	5.1	1¼
Stock gel (stock pots, stock melts and squeezy tubes)	5.7	1½	N	N	N	28g each	1.6	½
Stock, chicken, ready made, retail	0.1	0.0	N	N	N	50g	0.1	0
Stuffing mix, dried	4.4	1	2.0	1.6	0.8	1 whole (85g) packet	3.7	1
Stuffing mix, dried, assorted flavours, made up	1.3	¼	0.6	0.5	0.2	1 whole (85g) packet	1.1	¼
Stuffing, sage and onion, homemade	5.4	1¼	1.4	1.3	1.5	50g	2.7	¾
Suet, shredded	0.2	0	Tr	0.1	0.1	1 oz (28g)	0.1	0
Suet, vegetable, reduced fat	1.4	¼	Tr	0.7	0.7	1 oz (28g)	0.4	0
Sugar, brown	101.3	25¼	101.3	0.0	0.0	1 level teaspoon (4g)	4.1	1
Sugar, Demerara	104.5	26¼	104.5	0.0	0.0	1 level teaspoon (4g)	4.2	1
Sugar, icing	103.8	26	103.8	0.0	0.0	1 level teaspoon (4g)	4.2	1
Sugar, white	105.0	26¼	105.0	0.0	0.0	1 level teaspoon (4g)	4.2	1
Syrup, corn, dark	28.1	6	2.2	1.2	14.9	1 heaped teaspoon (17g)	4.8	1¼
						1 level teaspoon (8g)	2.2	½
Syrup, golden	79.0	19¾	32.8	23.0	23.1	1 heaped teaspoon (17g)	13.4	3¼
						1 level teaspoon (8g)	6.3	1½
						average spreading on 1 slice bread (20g)	15.8	4
Syrup, maple	60.7	15¼	56.5	1.1	3.1	serving on waffles (55g)	33.4	8¼
						1 heaped teaspoon (17g)	10.3	2½
						1 level teaspoon (8g)	4.9	1¼

Food name	Total sugars (g/100g)	Teaspoons (tsp) sugar/100g	Sucrose (g/100g)	Fructose (g/100g)	Glucose (g/100g)	Average portion size	Grams (g) sugar per average portion	Tsp sugar per average portion
Tahini paste	0.4	0	0.2	0.1	0.1	1 heaped teaspoon (19g)	0.1	0
Tomato puree	12.9	3¼	Tr	7.4	5.5	1 tablespoon (15g)	1.9	½
Treacle, black	66.8	16¾	32.7	16.7	17.4	1 heaped teaspoon (17g)	11.4	2¾
						1 level teaspoon (8g)	5.3	1¼
Whey, dried	78.0	19½	0.0	0.0	0.0	2 heaped scoops (45g)	35.1	8¾
Yeast, dried	Tr	0	Tr	Tr	Tr	1 7g sachet	Tr	0
Yeast extract	1.6	½	0.2	1.5	Tr	1 heaped teaspoon (18g)	0.3	0
						1 level teaspoon (9g)	0.1	0

Eggs and egg dishes

Food name

Food name	Total sugars (g/100g)	Teaspoons (tsp) sugar/100g	Sucrose (g/100g)	Fructose (g/100g)	Glucose (g/100g)	Average portion size	Grams (g) sugar per average portion	Tsp sugar per average portion
Curry, egg and potato, homemade	1.5	½	0.4	0.5	0.6	3–4 tablespoons (200g)	3	¾
Curry, egg, in sweet sauce, UK type, homemade	3.4	¾	0.5	1.5	1.3	3–4 tablespoons (200g)	6.8	1¾
Curry, egg, with butter, homemade (Punjabi dish)	3.4	¾	0.9	1.1	1.3	3–4 tablespoons (200g)	6.8	1¾
Curry, egg, with rapeseed oil, homemade (Punjabi dish)	3.3	¾	0.9	1.1	1.3	3–4 tablespoons (200g)	6.6	1¾
Eggs, chicken, scrambled, with semi-skimmed milk	0.7	¼	Tr	Tr	Tr	120g (2 eggs)	0.8	¼
Eggs, chicken, whole, boiled	Tr	0	0.0	0.0	Tr	average size (50g)	Tr	0
Eggs, chicken, whole, dried	Tr	0	0.0	0.0	Tr	1 tablespoon (5g)	0	0
Eggs, chicken, whole, fried	Tr	0	0.0	0.0	Tr	60g	Tr	0
Eggs, chicken, whole, poached	Tr	0	0.0	0.0	Tr	50g	Tr	0
Eggs, chicken, whole, raw	Tr	0	0.0	0.0	Tr	average size (50g)	Tr	0
Eggs, chicken, whole, scrambled, without milk	Tr	0	0.0	0.0	Tr	120g (2 eggs)	Tr	0
Eggs, duck, whole	Tr	0	0.0	0.0	Tr	75g each	Tr	0
Eggs, quail, whole	Tr	0	0.0	0.0	Tr	9g each	0	0
Eggs, turkey, whole	Tr	0	0.0	0.0	Tr	66g each	Tr	0
Egg fu yung	1.9	½	0.7	0.6	0.6	310g	5.9	1½
Omelette, cheese, homemade	Tr	0	0.0	0.0	Tr	150g (2 eggs)	Tr	0
Omelette, curried, homemade	1.4	¼	0.4	0.3	0.5	135g (2 eggs)	1.9	½
Omelette, plain, homemade	Tr	0	0.0	0.0	Tr	120g (2 eggs)	Tr	0
Omelette, Spanish, homemade	3.2	¾	1.0	1.1	1.1	260g	8.3	2
Potatoes with onions and eggs, fried (Greek dish)	1.4	¼	0.5	0.4	0.5	340g	4.8	1¼
Souffle, cheese, homemade	2.3	½	0.0	Tr	Tr	113g	2.6	¾
Souffle, plain, homemade	2.5	¾	0.0	Tr	Tr	113g	2.8	¾

Fats and oils

As you can see, most fats and
oils have no sugar at all.

Food name	Total sugars (g/100g)	Teaspoons (tsp) sugar/100g	Sucrose (g/100g)	Fructose (g/100g)	Glucose (g/100g)	Average portion size	Grams (g) sugar per average portion	Tsp sugar per average
Baking fat and margarine (75–90% fat), hard block (e.g. Stork)	0.0	0	0.0	0.0	0.0	1 teaspoon (5g)	0	0
Butter	0.6	¼	0.0	0.0	0.0	average spread on slice of bread: thin (7g),	0.0	0
						medium (10g),	0.1	0
						thick (12g)	0.1	0
						average spread on toasted crumpet (15g)	0.1	0
						1 curl (8g)	0.0	0
						1 portion pack (10g)	0.1	0
						1 teaspoon (5g)	0.0	0
Butter, spreadable (75–80% fat)	0.5	¼	0.0	0.0	0.0	average spread on slice of bread: thin (7g),	0.0	0
						medium (10g),	0.1	0
						thick (12g)	0.1	0
						average spread on toasted crumpet (15g)	0.1	0
						1 curl (8g)	0.1	0
						1 portion pack (10g)	0.1	0
						1 teaspoon (5g)	0.0	
Butter, spreadable, light (60% fat)	0.8	¼	0.0	0.0	0.0	average spread on slice of bread: thin (7g),	0.0	0
						medium (10g),	0.1	0
						thick (12g)	0.1	0
						average spread on toasted crumpet (15g)	0.1	0
						1 curl (8g)	0.1	0
						1 portion pack (10g)	0.1	0
						1 teaspoon (5g)	0.0	0
Butteroil	Tr	0	0.0	0.0	0.0	1 tablespoon (13g)	0	0
Dripping, beef	0.0	0	0.0	0.0	0.0	1 tablespoon (13g)	0	0
Fat spread (20–25% fat), not polyunsaturated	1.1	¼	0.0	0.0	0.0	average spread on slice of bread: thin (5g),	0.1	0
						medium (7g),	0.1	0
						thick (10g)	0.1	0
						average spread on toasted crumpet (10g)	0.1	0
						thin scraping on crisp bread (2g)	0.0	0
						1 portion pack (10g)	0.1	0
						1 teaspoon (5g)	0.1	0

Food name	Total sugars (g/100g)	Teaspoons (tsp) sugar/100g	Sucrose (g/100g)	Fructose (g/100g)	Glucose (g/100g)	Average portion size	Grams (g) sugar per average portion	Tsp sugar per average portion
Fat spread (20–25% fat), polyunsaturated	0.0	0	0.0	0.0	0.0	average spread on slice of bread: thin (5g),	0.0	0
						medium (7g),	0.0	0
						thick (10g)	0.0	0
						average spread on toasted crumpet (10g)	0.0	0
						thin scraping on crisp bread (2g)	0.0	0
						1 portion pack (10g)	0.0	0
						1 teaspoon (5g)	0.0	0
Fat spread, low fat (26–39%), not polyunsaturated, including dairy type	0.4	0	0.0	0.0	0.0	average spread on slice of bread: thin (5g),	0.0	0
						medium (7g),	0.0	0
						thick (10g)	0.0	0
						average spread on toasted crumpet (10g)	0.0	0
						thin scraping on crisp bread (2g)	0.0	0
						1 portion pack (10g)	0.0	0
						1 teaspoon (5g)	0.0	0
Fat spread, low fat (26–39%), not polyunsaturated, with olive oil	0.5	¼	0.0	0.0	0.0	average spread on slice of bread: thin (5g),	0.1	0
						medium (7g),	0.1	0
						thick (10g)	0.1	0
						average spread on toasted crumpet (10g)	0.1	0
						thin scraping on crisp bread (2g)	0.0	0
						1 portion pack (10g)	0.1	0
						1 teaspoon (5g)	0.1	0
Fat spread, low fat (26–39%), polyunsaturated	1.3	0.3	0.0	0.0	0.0	average spread on slice of bread: thin (5g),	0.1	0
						medium (7g),	0.1	0
						thick (10g)	0.1	0
						average spread on toasted crumpet (10g)	0.0	0
						thin scraping on crisp bread (2g)	0.1	0
						1 portion pack (10g)	0.1	0
						1 teaspoon (5g)		0
Fat spread, reduced fat (41–62%), not polyunsaturated	1.3	0.3	0.0	0.0	0.0	average spread on slice of bread: thin (5g),	0.1	0
						medium (7g),	0.1	0
						thick (10g)	0.1	0
						average spread on toasted crumpet (10g)	0.0	0
						thin scraping on crisp bread (2g)	0.1	0
						1 portion pack (10g)	0.1	0
						1 teaspoon (5g)	0.1	0

Food name	Total sugars (g/100g)	Teaspoons (tsp) sugar/100g	Sucrose (g/100g)	Fructose (g/100g)	Glucose (g/100g)	Average portion size	Grams (g) sugar per average portion	Tsp sugar per average portion
Fat spread, reduced fat (41–62%), not polyunsaturated, with olive oil	1.1	¼	0.0	0.0	0.0	average spread on slice of bread: thin (5g),	0.1	0
						medium (7g),	0.1	0
						thick (10g)	0.1	0
						average spread on toasted crumpet (10g)	0.1	0
						thin scraping on crisp bread (2g)	0.0	0
						1 portion pack (10g)	0.1	0
						1 teaspoon (5g)	0.1	0
Fat spread, reduced fat (41–62%), polyunsaturated	Tr	0	0.0	0.0	0.0	average spread on slice of bread: thin (5g),	0.0	0
						medium (7g),	0.0	0
						thick (10g)	0.0	0
						average spread on toasted crumpet (10g)	0.0	0
						thin scraping on crisp bread (2g)	0.0	0
						1 portion pack (10g)	0.0	0
						1 teaspoon (5g)	0.0	0
Fat spread, reduced fat (62–75%), not polyunsaturated	Tr	0	0.0	0.0	0.0	average spread on slice of bread: thin (5g),	0.0	0
						medium (7g),	0.0	0
						thick (10g)	0.0	0
						average spread on toasted crumpet (10g)	0.0	0
						thin scraping on crisp bread (2g)	0.0	0
						1 portion pack (10g)	0.0	0
						1 teaspoon (5g)	0.0	0
Fat spread, reduced fat (62–75%), polyunsaturated	0.6	¼	0.0	0.0	0.0	average spread on slice of bread: thin (5g),	0.0	0
						medium (7g),	0.1	0
						thick (10g)	0.1	0
						average spread on toasted crumpet (10g)	0.1	0
						thin scraping on crisp bread (2g)	0.0	0
						1 portion pack (10g)	0.1	0
						1 teaspoon (5g)	0.0	0
Ghee made from butter	Tr	0	0.0	0.0	0.0	1 teaspoon (5g)	0.0	0
Lard	0.0	0	0.0	0.0	0.0	1 tablespoon (13g)	0.0	0
Oil, blackcurrant seed	0.0	0	0.0	0.0	0.0	1 tablespoon (11g)	0.0	0
						1 teaspoon (3g)	0.0	0
Oil, borage	0.0	0	0.0	0.0	0.0	1 tablespoon (11g)	0.0	0
						1 teaspoon (3g)	0.0	0

Food name	Total sugars (g/100g)	Teaspoons (tsp) sugar/100g	Sucrose (g/100g)	Fructose (g/100g)	Glucose (g/100g)	Average portion size	Grams (g) sugar per average portion	Tsp sugar per average portion
Oil, coconut	0.0	0	0.0	0.0	0.0	1 tablespoon (11g)	0.0	0
						1 teaspoon (3g)	0.0	0
Oil, cod liver	0.0	0	0.0	0.0	0.0	1 tablespoon (11g)	0.0	0
						1 teaspoon (3g)	0.0	0
Oil, corn	0.0	0	0.0	0.0	0.0	1 tablespoon (11g)	0.0	0
						1 teaspoon (3g)	0.0	0
Oil, cottonseed	0.0	0	0.0	0.0	0.0	1 tablespoon (11g)	0.0	0
						1 teaspoon (3g)	0.0	0
Oil, evening primrose	0.0	0	0.0	0.0	0.0	1 tablespoon (11g)	0.0	0
						1 teaspoon (3g)	0.0	0
Oil, grapeseed	0.0	0	0.0	0.0	0.0	1 tablespoon (11g)	0.0	0
						1 teaspoon (3g)	0.0	0
Oil, hazelnut	0.0	0	0.0	0.0	0.0	1 tablespoon (11g)	0.0	0
						1 teaspoon (3g)	0.0	0
Oil, olive	0.0	0	0.0	0.0	0.0	1 tablespoon (11g)	0.0	0
						1 teaspoon (3g)	0.0	0
Oil, palm	0.0	0	0.0	0.0	0.0	1 tablespoon (11g)	0.0	0
						1 teaspoon (3g)	0.0	0
Oil, peanut (groundnut)	0.0	0	0.0	0.0	0.0	1 tablespoon (11g)	0.0	0
						1 teaspoon (3g)	0.0	0
Oil, rapeseed	0.0	0	0.0	0.0	0.0	1 tablespoon (11g)	0.0	0
						1 teaspoon (3g)	0.0	0
Oil, safflower	0.0	0	0.0	0.0	0.0	1 tablespoon (11g)	0.0	0
						1 teaspoon (3g)	0.0	0
Oil, sesame	0.0	0	0.0	0.0	0.0	1 tablespoon (11g)	0.0	0
						1 teaspoon (3g)	0.0	0
Oil, soya	0.0	0	0.0	0.0	0.0	1 tablespoon (11g)	0.0	0
						1 teaspoon (3g)	0.0	0
Oil, sunflower	0.0	0	0.0	0.0	0.0	1 tablespoon (11g)	0.0	0
						1 teaspoon (3g)	0.0	0
Oil, vegetable	0.0	0	0.0	0.0	0.0	1 tablespoon (11g)	0.0	0
						1 teaspoon (3g)	0.0	0
Oil, walnut	0.0	0	0.0	0.0	0.0	1 tablespoon (11g)	0.0	0
						1 teaspoon (3g)	0.0	0
Oil, wheatgerm	0.0	0	0.0	0.0	0.0	1 tablespoon (11g)	0.0	0
						1 teaspoon (3g)	0.0	0

Fish, fish dishes and seafood

Food name	Total sugars (g/100g)	Teaspoons (tsp) sugar/100g	Sucrose (g/100g)	Fructose (g/100g)	Glucose (g/100g)	Average portion size	Grams (g) sugar per average portion	Tsp sugar per average portion
Abalone, canned in brine, drained	Tr	0	0.0	0.0	0.0	small jar (155g)	Tr	0
Anchovies, canned in oil, drained	0.0	0	0.0	0.0	0.0	1 anchovy (3g)	0	0
Bass, sea, flesh only, baked	0.0	0	0.0	0.0	0.0	90g per fillet	0	0
Bele raw (scribbled goby fish)	0.0	0	0.0	0.0	0.0	small portion (100g) medium portion (150g) large portion (180g)	0.0 0.0 0.0	0 0 0
Bloater, flesh only	0.0	0	0.0	0.0	0.0	small portion (100g) medium portion (150g) large portion (180g)	0.0 0.0 0.0	0 0 0
Boal, raw	0.0	0	0.0	0.0	0.0	small portion (100g) medium portion (150g) large portion (180g)	0.0 0.0 0.0	0 0 0
Bombay duck	0.0	0	0.0	0.0	0.0	1 small fresh fish (115g)	0	0
Bream, Sea, raw	0.0	0	0.0	0.0	0.0	small portion (100g) medium portion (150g) large portion (180g)	0.0 0.0 0.0	0 0 0
Calamari, coated in batter, baked	Tr	0	Tr	Tr	Tr	1 average portion (120g)	Tr	0
Carp, raw	0.0	0	0.0	0.0	0.0	small portion (100g) medium portion (150g) large portion (180g)	0.0 0.0 0.0	0 0 0
Catfish, flesh only, steamed	0.0	0	0.0	0.0	0.0	small portion (100g) medium portion (150g) large portion (180g)	0.0 0.0 0.0	0 0 0
Caviare, bottled in brine, drained	0.0	0	0.0	0.0	0.0	1 tablespoon (19g)	0	0
Clams, canned in brine, drained	Tr	0	0.0	0.0	0.0	small jar (155g)	Tr	0
Cockles, boiled	Tr	0	0.0	0.0	0.0	1 cockle (4g)	0	0
Cockles, bottled in vinegar, drained	Tr	0	0.0	0.0	0.0	small jar (142g)	Tr	0
Cod, baked, grilled, steamed or microwaved	0.0	0	0.0	0.0	0.0	small fillet (50g) medium fillet (120g) large fillet (175g)	0.0 0.0 0.0	0 0 0
Cod, poached in milk	Tr	0	0.0	0.0	0.0	small fillet (50g) medium fillet (120g) large fillet (175g)	0.0 Tr Tr	0 0 0

Food name	Total sugars (g/100g)	Teaspoons (tsp) sugar/100g	Sucrose (g/100g)	Fructose (g/100g)	Glucose (g/100g)	Average portion size	Grams (g) sugar per average portion	Tsp sugar per average portion
Cod, flesh only, salted and smoked, raw	0.0	0	0.0	0.0	0.0	small fillet (50g) medium fillet (120g) large fillet (175g)	0.0 0.0 0.0	0 0 0
Cod, in batter, baked	2.0	½	N	Tr	N	small (120g) medium (180g) large (225g)	2.4 3.6 4.5	½ 1 1
Cod, in batter, fried	1.0	¼	0.3	0.2	0.1	small (120g) medium (180g) large (225g)	1.2 1.8 2.3	¼ ½ ½
Cod, in breadcrumbs, baked	0.9	¼	0.1	Tr	0.2	100g	0.9	¼
Cod, in parsley sauce, frozen, boiled	Tr	0	Tr	Tr	Tr	170g	Tr	0
Coley, flesh only, cooked	0.0	0	0.0	0.0	0.0	small fillet (100g) medium fillet (150g) large filet (180g)	0.0 0.0 0.0	0 0 0
Crab, canned in brine, drained	Tr	0	0.0	0.0	0.0	1 small can (85g)	Tr	0
Crab, purchased cooked	Tr	0	0.0	0.0	0.0	1 dressed crab, no shell (130g) 1 tablespoon crab meat (40g)	Tr 0.0	0 0
Crayfish, raw, weighed with shell	0.0	0	0.0	0.0	0.0	1 small fish (100g)	0	0
Curry, fish and vegetable, Bangladeshi, homemade	1.1	¼	0.3	0.4	0.4	small portion (200g) medium portion (300g)	2.2 3.3	½ ¾
Curry, fish, Bangladeshi, homemade	1.2	¼	0.4	0.4	0.4	small portion (200g) medium portion (300g)	2.4 3.6	½ 1
Curry, fish, homemade	1.9	½	0.4	0.7	0.5	small portion (200g) medium portion (300g)	3.8 5.7	1 1 ½
Curry, haddock, Bengali, homemade	3.2	¾	0.8	1.0	1.2	small portion (200g) medium portion (300g)	6.4 9.6	1 ½ 2 ½
Curry, herring, Bengali, homemade	3.2	¾	0.8	1.0	1.2	small portion (200g) medium portion (300g)	6.4 9.6	1 ½ 2 ½
Curry, prawn and mushroom, homemade	1.7	½	0.5	0.6	0.7	small portion (200g) medium portion (300g)	3.4 5.1	¾ 1 ¼
Cuttlefish, raw	0.0	0	0.0	0.0	0.0	small portion (100g) medium portion (150g) large portion (180g)	0.0 0.0 0.0	0 0 0

Food name	Total sugars (g/100g)	Teaspoons (tsp) sugar/100g	Sucrose (g/100g)	Fructose (g/100g)	Glucose (g/100g)	Average portion size	Grams (g) sugar per average portion	Tsp sugar per average portion
Dab, raw	0.0	0	0.0	0.0	0.0	small portion (100g)	0.0	0
						medium portion (150g)	0.0	0
						large portion (180g)	0.0	0
Dover sole, raw	0.0	0	0.0	0.0	0.0	1 whole, with bone (250g)	0	0
Eel, grilled, flesh only	0.0	0	0.0	0.0	0.0	115g	0	0
Eel, grilled, weighed with bones and skin	0.0	0	0.0	0.0	0.0	225g	0	0
Eel, jellied	0.0	0	0.0	0.0	0.0	1 slice, 5'' long (20g)	0	0
Fish balls, steamed (Chinese dish)	Tr	0	0.0	0.0	0.0	150g	Tr	0
Fish fingers, cod, fried	1.3	¼	0.2	Tr	Tr	60g each	0.8	¼
Fish fingers, cod, grilled/baked	1.5	¼	0.2	Tr	Tr	60g each	0.9	¼
Fish fingers, pollock, grilled	1.3	¼	Tr	0.1	0.4	60g each	0.8	¼
Fish fingers, salmon, grilled/baked	1.1	¼	Tr	0.1	0.1	60g each	0.7	¼
Fish paste	0.5	0	0.5	Tr	Tr	average spread on a slice of bread (10g)	0.1	0
						as a starter (40g)	0.2	0
Fishcakes, cod, homemade	0.7	¼	0.1	0.1	0.1	135g each	0.9	¼
Fishcakes, salmon, coated in breadcrumbs, baked	1.6	½	Tr	0.2	0.1	135g each	2.2	½
Fishcakes, salmon, homemade	0.7	¼	0.1	0.1	0.1	135g each	0.9	¼
Fishcakes, white fish, coated in breadcrumbs, baked	1.8	½	0.1	0.2	0.2	135g each	2.4	½
Flounder, flesh only, steamed	0.0	0	0.0	0.0	0.0	small portion (100g)	0.0	0
						medium portion (150g)	0.0	0
						large portion (180g)	0.0	0
Flying fish, raw	0.0	0	0.0	0.0	0.0	small portion (100g)	0.0	0
						medium portion (150g)	0.0	0
						large portion (180g)	0.0	0
Haddock, coated in crumbs, frozen, fried	Tr	0	Tr	Tr	Tr	120g	Tr	0

Food name	Total sugars (g/100g)	Teaspoons (tsp) sugar/100g	Sucrose (g/100g)	Fructose (g/100g)	Glucose (g/100g)	Average portion size	Grams (g) sugar per average portion	Tsp sugar per average portion
Haddock, fillets, flesh only, in flour, fried	Tr	0	Tr	Tr	Tr	small fillet (50g) medium fillet (120g) large fillet (170g)	0.0 Tr Tr	0 0 0
Haddock, flesh only, grilled, poached or steamed	0.0	0	0.0	0.0	0.0	small fillet (50g) medium fillet (120g) large fillet (170g)	0.0 0.0 0.0	0 0 0
Haddock, in batter, fried	Tr	0	Tr	Tr	Tr	small fillet (120g) medium fillet (170g) large fillet (220g)	Tr Tr Tr	0 0 0
Hake, flesh only, grilled	0.0	0	0.0	0.0	0.0	1 average steak (100g)	0	0
Halibut, flesh only, grilled	0.0	0	0.0	0.0	0.0	1 average steak (145g)	0	0
Halibut, flesh only, poached	1.1	¼	0.0	0.0	0.0	110g	1.2	¼
Herring, canned in tomato sauce, whole contents	2.9	¾	1.1	1.0	0.8	1 can (200g)	5.8	1 ½
Herring, flesh only, grilled	0.0	0	0.0	0.0	0.0	small fillet (85g) medium fillet (119g)	0.0 0.0	0 0
Herring, pickled (rollmop)	10.0	2½	10.0	0.0	0.0	90g each	9	2¼
Hilsa, raw	0.0	0	0.0	0.0	0.0	small portion (100g) medium portion (150g) large portion (180g)	0.0 0.0 0.0	0 0 0
Hoki, grilled	0.0	0	0.0	0.0	0.0	1 average fillet (190g)	0	0
Jackfish, raw	0.0	0	0.0	0.0	0.0	small portion (100g) medium portion (150g) large portion (180g)	0.0 0.0 0.0	0 0 0
John Dory, raw	0.0	0	0.0	0.0	0.0	small portion (100g) medium portion (150g) large portion (180g)	0.0 0.0 0.0	0 0 0
Kalabasu, raw	0.0	0	0.0	0.0	0.0	small portion (100g) medium portion (150g) large portion (180g)	0.0 0.0 0.0	0 0 0
Katla, raw	0.0	0	0.0	0.0	0.0	small portion (100g) medium portion (150g) large portion (180g)	0.0 0.0 0.0	0 0 0
Kedgeree, homemade	Tr	0	Tr	Tr	Tr	300g	Tr	0
Kippers, flesh only, boil in the bag, with butter, cooked	Tr	0	0.0	0.0	0.0	170g	Tr	0

Food name	Total sugars (g/100g)	Teaspoons (tsp) sugar/100g	Sucrose (g/100g)	Fructose (g/100g)	Glucose (g/100g)	Average portion size	Grams (g) sugar per average portion	Tsp sugar per average portion
Kippers, grilled	0.0	0	0.0	0.0	0.0	small fillet (85g)	0.0	0
						medium fillet (130g)	0.0	0
						large fillet (170g)	0.0	0
Langoustine, boiled, weighed with shells	0.0	0	0.0	0.0	0.0	250g	0	0
Lemon sole, grilled or steamed	0.0	0	0.0	0.0	0.0	small fillet (100g)	0.0	0
						medium fillet (170g)	0.0	0
						large fillet (220g)	0.0	0
Lemon sole, goujons, baked	0.9	¼	Tr	Tr	Tr	15g per goujon	0.1	0
Ling, raw	0.0	0	0.0	0.0	0.0	small portion (100g)	0.0	0
						medium portion (150g)	0.0	0
						large portion (180g)	0.0	0
Lobster, boiled	Tr	0	0.0	0.0	0.0	2 tablespoon (85g)	Tr	0
Lobster, boiled, weighed with shell	Tr	0	0.0	0.0	0.0	half dressed lobster (250g)	Tr	0
Mackerel, canned in oil	0.0	0	0.0	0.0	0.0	200g per can	0	0
Mackerel, canned in tomato sauce, whole contents	1.4	¼	0.3	0.6	0.5	125g per can	1.75	½
Mackerel, flesh only, grilled or fried	0.0	0	0.0	0.0	0.0	1 whole fish (220g)	0	0
Mackerel, flesh only, smoked	0.0	0	0.0	0.0	0.0	1 small fish (100g)	0.0	0
						1 medium fish (150g)	0.0	0
						1 large fish (200g)	0.0	0
Monkfish, flesh only, grilled	0.0	0	0.0	0.0	0.0	70g	0	0
Mullet, Grey, flesh only, grilled	0.0	0	0.0	0.0	0.0	100g	0	0
Mullet, Grey, grilled, weighed with bones and skin	0.0	0	0.0	0.0	0.0	small portion (100g)	0.0	0
						medium portion (150g)	0.0	0
						large portion (180g)	0.0	0
Mullet, Red, flesh only, grilled	0.0	0	0.0	0.0	0.0	1 average whole (75g)	0	0
Mussels, canned and bottled, drained	Tr	0	0.0	0.0	0.0	small jar (80g)	Tr	0
Mussels in white wine sauce, cooked	0.8	¼	0.0	0.0	0.0	40g (no shells)	0.3	0
Mussels, purchased cooked	Tr	0	0.0	0.0	0.0	7g each (no shell)	0	0

Food name	Total sugars (g/100g)	Teaspoons (tsp) sugar/100g	Sucrose (g/100g)	Fructose (g/100g)	Glucose (g/100g)	Average portion size	Grams (g) sugar per average portion	Tsp sugar per average portion
Octopus, raw	Tr	0	0.0	0.0	0.0	average portion (100g)	Tr	0
Orange Roughy, raw	0.0	0	0.0	0.0	0.0	small portion (100g)	0.0	0
						medium portion (150g)	0.0	0
						large portion (180g)	0.0	0
Oysters, raw	Tr	0	0.0	0.0	0.0	10g each (no shell)	0	0
Pangasius (River Cobbler), flesh only, baked or poached	0.0	0	0.0	0.0	0.0	small portion (100g)	0.0	0
						medium portion (150g)	0.0	0
						large portion (180g)	0.0	0
Parrot fish, raw	0.0	0	0.0	0.0	0.0	small portion (100g)	0.0	0
						medium portion (150g)	0.0	0
						large portion (180g)	0.0	0
Pate, mackerel, smoked	0.7	¼	Tr	Tr	0.1	average spread on a slice of bread (10g)	0.0	0
						as a starter (40g)	0.3	0
Pate, tuna	0.4	0	0.2	0.1	0.1	average spread on a slice of bread (10g)	0.0	0
						as a starter (40g)	0.2	0
Pilchards, canned in tomato sauce, whole contents	0.9	¼	Tr	0.5	0.4	small can (215g)	1.9	½
Plaice, flesh only, baked or steamed	0.0	0	0.0	0.0	0.0	small fillet (75g)	0.0	0
						medium fillet (130g)	0.0	0
						large fillet (180g)	0.0	0
Plaice, in batter, fried	Tr	0	Tr	Tr	Tr	small fillet (150g)	Tr	0
						medium fillet (200g)	Tr	0
						large fillet (250g)	Tr	0
Plaice, in breadcrumbs, baked	1.3	¼	Tr	Tr	0.2	small fillet (90g)	1.2	¼
						medium fillet (150g)	2.0	½
						large fillet (200g)	2.6	¾
Pollock, Alaskan, flesh only	0.0	0	0.0	0.0	0.0	small portion (100g)	0.0	0
						medium portion (150g)	0.0	0
						large portion (180g)	0.0	0
Pomfret, raw	0.0	0	0.0	0.0	0.0	small portion (100g)	0.0	0
						medium portion (150g)	0.0	0
						large portion (180g)	0.0	0
Prawns, king, cooked, no shell	0.0	0	0.0	0.0	0.0	8g each	0	0
Prawns, standard, purchased cooked, weighed with shells	0.0	0	0.0	0.0	0.0	3g each (no shell)	0.0	0
						half a pint, shelled (142g)	0.0	0
Red snapper, flesh only, fried	0.0	0	0.0	0.0	0.0	1 average whole (200g)	0	0

Food name	Total sugars (g/100g)	Teaspoons (tsp) sugar/100g	Sucrose (g/100g)	Fructose (g/100g)	Glucose (g/100g)	Average portion size	Grams (g) sugar per average portion	Tsp sugar per average
Redfish, raw	0.0	0	0.0	0.0	0.0	small portion (100g) medium portion (150g) large portion (180g)	0.0 0.0 0.0	0 0 0
Rock Salmon/Dogfish, in batter, fried	Tr	0	Tr	Tr	Tr	small portion (150g) medium portion (200g) large portion (250g)	Tr Tr Tr	0 0 0
Roe, cod, hard, coated in batter, fried	Tr	0	Tr	Tr	Tr	160g	Tr	0
Roe, cod, hard, raw	0.0	0	0.0	0.0	0.0	116g	0	0
Roe, herring, soft, raw	0.0	0	0.0	0.0	0.0	85g	0	0
Rohu, raw	0.0	0	0.0	0.0	0.0	small portion (100g) medium portion (150g) large portion (180g)	0.0 0.0 0.0	0 0 0
Salmon en croute, retail	0.9	¼	0.1	Tr	0.1	190g per steak	1.7	½
Salmon, flesh only, baked, grilled or steamed	0.0	0	0.0	0.0	0.0	1 average steak (100g) 1 large steak (170g)	0.0 0.0	0 0
Salmon, canned in brine, drained	0.0	0	0.0	0.0	0.0	1 portion (100g) in a sandwich (45g)	0.0 0.0	0 0
Salmon, smoked (cold-smoked)	0.5	0	Tr	Tr	Tr	56g	0.3	0
Salmon, smoked (hot-smoked)	1.3	¼	0.8	Tr	Tr	56g	0.7	¼
Salted fish, Chinese, bones removed, steamed	0.0	0	0.0	0.0	0.0	small portion (100g) medium portion (150g) large portion (180g)	0.0 0.0 0.0	0 0 0
Sardines, canned in oil, drained	0.0	0	0.0	0.0	0.0	1 sardine (25g) 1 can (100g)	0.0 0.0	0 0
Sardines, canned in tomato sauce, whole contents	0.9	¼	Tr	0.6	0.3	1 sardine (25g) 1 can (100g)	0.2 0.9	0 0
Sardines, flesh only, grilled	0.0	0	0.0	0.0	0.0	6 sardines (86g)	0	0
Scallops, steamed	Tr	0	0.0	0.0	0.0	90g	Tr	0
Scampi, coated in breadcrumbs, baked	0.8	¼	Tr	Tr	Tr	1 piece of scampi (15g) 1 average portion (170g)	0.1 1.4	0 ¼
Scampi, coated in breadcrumbs, fried	0.7	¼	Tr	Tr	Tr	1 piece of scampi (15g) 1 average portion (170g)	0.1 1.2	 ¼
Seafood pasta, retail	1.6	½	0.1	0.2	0.2	235g	3.8	1

Food name	Total sugars (g/100g)	Teaspoons (tsp) sugar/100g	Sucrose (g/100g)	Fructose (g/100g)	Glucose (g/100g)	Average portion size	Grams (g) sugar per average portion	Tsp sugar per average portion
Seafood selection (mussels, prawns, squid and cockles)	Tr	0	0.0	0.0	0.0	110g	Tr	0
Seafood sticks	4.8	1¼	4.8	Tr	Tr	17g per stick	0.8	¼
Shark, raw	0.0	0	0.0	0.0	0.0	small portion (100g)	0.0	0
						medium portion (150g)	0.0	0
						large portion (180g)	0.0	0
Shrimps, boiled, weighed without shells	Tr	0	0.0	0.0	0.0	50g	Tr	0
Shrimps, canned in brine, drained	Tr	0	0.0	0.0	0.0	90g pack	Tr	0
Shrimps, dried	Tr	0	0.0	0.0	0.0	1oz (28g)	0	0
Shrimps, frozen, weighed with shells	Tr	0	0.0	0.0	0.0	150g	Tr	0
Skate, grilled	0.0	0	0.0	0.0	0.0	1 average large wing (290g)	0	0
Sole, flesh only, grilled, fillets weighed with skin	0.0	0	0.0	0.0	0.0	120g per fillet	0	0
Sprats, fried	0.0	0	0.0	0.0	0.0	1 sprat (55g)	0.0	0
						1 average portion (220g)	0.0	0
Squid, cooked	Tr	0	0.0	0.0	0.0	1 average portion (65g)	Tr	0
Sushi, salmon nigiri	3.2	¾	1.5	0.5	0.5	17g per piece	0.5	0
Sushi, tuna nigiri	4.7	1¼	2.2	0.5	1.0	17g per piece	0.8	¼
Sushi, vegetable	7.0	1¾	0.5	2.4	2.5	17g per piece	1.2	¼
Swordfish, flesh only, grilled	0.0	0	0.0	0.0	0.0	1 average portion (140g)	0	0
Tilapia, raw	0.0	0	0.0	0.0	0.0	small portion (100g)	0.0	0
						medium portion (150g)	0.0	0
						large portion (180g)	0.0	0
Trout, brown, steamed, weighed without bones and head	0.0	0				1 average trout (155g)	0	0
Trout, brown, steamed, weighed with bones and head	0.0	0				1 average trout (230g)	0	0
Trout, rainbow, flesh only, baked	0.0	0	0.0	0.0	0.0	155g (without bones and head)	0	0
Tuna, canned in brine, drained	0.0	0	0.0	0.0	0.0	1 small can (100g)	0.0	0
						in a sandwich (45g)	0.0	0

Food name	Total sugars (g/100g)	Teaspoons (tsp) sugar/100g	Sucrose (g/100g)	Fructose (g/100g)	Glucose (g/100g)	Average portion size	Grams (g) sugar per average portion	Tsp sugar per average portion
Tuna, canned in sunflower oil, drained	0.0	0	0.0	0.0	0.0	1 small can (100g) in a sandwich (45g)	0.0 0.0	0 0
Tuna, flesh only, baked	0.0	0	0.0	0.0	0.0	125g per steak	0	0
Turbot, flesh only, grilled	0.0	0	0.0	0.0	0.0	1 average whole (160g)	0	0
Whelks, boiled, weighed without shells	Tr	0	0.0	0.0	0.0	1 whelk (7g)	0	0
Whelks, boiled, weighed with shells	Tr	0	0.0	0.0	0.0	1 average portion (30g)	0	0
White fish, dried, salted	0.0	0	0.0	0.0	0.0	small fillet (100g) medium fillet (150g) large filet (180g)	0.0 0.0 0.0	0 0 0
Whitebait, in flour, fried	0.1	0	Tr	Tr	Tr	1 whitebait (4g) 1 average portion (80g)	0.0 0.0	0 0
Whiting, flesh only, steamed, weighed without bones and skin	0.0	0	0.0	0.0	0.0	85g	0	0
Whiting, in crumbs, fried, weighed with bones and skin	0.2	0	Tr	Tr	Tr	small fillet (120g) medium fillet (180g) large fillet (240g)	0.2 0.4 0.5	0 0 0
Winkles, boiled	Tr	0	0.0	0.0	0.0	1 average portion (30g)	0	0

Fruit – fresh, dried, stewed and tinned

Food name	Total sugars (g/100g)	Teaspoons (tsp) sugar/100g	Sucrose (g/100g)	Fructose (g/100g)	Glucose (g/100g)	Average portion size	Grams (g) sugar per average portion	Tsp sugar per average
Acca (feijoa), flesh only	10.0	2½	N	N	N	85g each	8.5	2
Ackee, canned, drained	0.8	¼	0.7	Tr	0.1	½ 540g can (270g)	2.2	½
Apples, cooking, baked with sugar, flesh only, weighed with skin	14.3	3½	6.8	5.5	2.0	190g	27.2	6¾
Apples, cooking, baked without sugar, flesh only, weighed with skin	9.6	2½	1.6	5.9	2.1	190g	18.2	2½
Apples, cooking, raw, flesh only, weighed with skin and core	6.4	1½	0.7	4.3	1.5	190g	12.2	3
Apples, cooking, stewed with sugar, flesh only	20.8	5¼	11.0	6.7	3.1	110g	22.9	5¾
Apples, cooking, stewed without sugar, flesh only	9.7	1½	1.7	5.9	2.1	85g	8.2	2
Apples, eating, dried	60.1	15	19.9	31.7	8.6	½ of a 120g packet (60g)	36.1	9
Apples, eating, raw, flesh and skin, weighed with core	10.0	2½	2.4	5.8	1.8	small (75g) medium (112g) large (170g)	7.5 11.2 17.0	1¾ 2¾ 4¼
Apricots, canned in juice, whole contents	8.4	2	1.4	4.1	3.0	140g	11.8	3
Apricots, canned in syrup, whole contents	16.1	4	3.7	5.8	6.7	140g	22.5	5½
Apricots, dried	43.4	10¾	12.6	10.0	20.8	1 fruit (8g)	3.5	¾
Apricots, dried, stewed with sugar	22.0	5½	8.9	4.4	8.7	140g	30.8	7¾
Apricots, dried, stewed without sugar	17.8	4½	4.7	4.4	8.8	140g	24.9	6¼
Apricots, raw, flesh and skin, weighed without stone	7.2	1¾	4.6	0.9	1.6	1 fruit (40g)	2.9	¾
Apricots, ready-to-eat, semi-dried	36.5	9	10.6	8.4	17.5	1 fruit (9g)	3.3	¾
Apricots, stewed with sugar, weighed without stones	18.3	4½	14.0	2.1	2.2	140g	25.6	6½
Apricots, stewed without sugar, weighed without stones	6.2	1½	3.5	1.0	1.6	140g	8.7	2¼

Food name	Total sugars (g/100g)	Teaspoons (tsp) sugar/100g	Sucrose (g/100g)	Fructose (g/100g)	Glucose (g/100g)	Average portion size	Grams (g) sugar per average portion	Tsp sugar per average portion
Babaco, flesh only	3.1	¾	0.7	1.1	1.3	1 whole small fruit (454g)	14.1	3½
						1 whole large fruit (907g)	28.2	7
Banana chips, crystallised	22.1	5½	21.7	0.3	0.1	10 chips (13g)	2.9	¾
Bananas, flesh only, weighed without skin	18.1	4½	2.7	7.5	7.9	1 small (80g)	14.5	3½
						1 medium (100g)	18.1	4½
						1 large (120g)	21.7	5½
Blackberries, raw	5.1	1¼	Tr	2.6	2.5	5g each	0.3	0
Blackberries, stewed with sugar	13.8	3½	8.9	2.5	2.5	140g	19.3	4¾
Blackberries, stewed without sugar	4.4	1	Tr	2.2	2.1	140g	6.2	1½
Blackberry and apple, stewed with sugar	15.8	4	10.5	3.6	1.7	140g	22.1	5½
Blackberry and apple, stewed without sugar	6.4	1½	0.5	3.9	1.9	140g	9	2¼
Blackcurrants, canned in juice, whole contents	7.6	2	0.2	4.0	3.4	½ can (145g)	11	2¾
Blackcurrants, canned in syrup, whole contents	18.4	4½	2.0	8.3	8.1	½ can (145g)	26.7	7¾
Blackcurrants, raw	6.6	1¾	0.3	3.4	3.0	5 currants (2g)	0.1	0
Blackcurrants, stewed with sugar	15.0	3¾	9.0	3.2	2.8	140g	21	5¼
Blackcurrants, stewed without sugar	5.6	1½	0.2	2.9	2.5	140g	7.8	2
Blueberries	9.1	1¼	Tr	5.2	3.9	2g each	0.2	0
Boysenberries, canned in syrup, whole contents	20.4	5	N	N	N	½ 425g can (213g)	43.5	10¾
Breadfruit, boiled in water	1.5	½	N	N	N	140g	2.1	½
Breadfruit, canned, drained	1.8	½	N	N	N	½ 538g can (269g)	4.8	1¼
Breadfruit, raw	1.2	¼	N	N	N	1 small fruit (300g)	3.6	1
Cashew fruit, flesh only	6.8	1¾	N	N	N	1 whole fruit (56g)	3.8	1
Cherries, canned in syrup, whole contents	18.5	4¾	4.3	6.6	7.3	½ can (215g)	39.8	10
Cherries, flesh and skin, raw, weighed without stone	11.5	3	0.2	5.3	5.9	4g each	0.5	0

Food name	Total sugars (g/100g)	Teaspoons (tsp) sugar/100g	Sucrose (g/100g)	Fructose (g/100g)	Glucose (g/100g)	Average portion size	Grams (g) sugar per average portion	Tsp sugar per average portion
Cherries, stewed with sugar, weighed without stones	21.0	5¼	10.9	4.8	5.2	140g	29.4	7½
Cherries, stewed without sugar, weighed without stones	10.1	2½	0.2	4.7	5.2	140g	14.1	3½
Cherries, West Indian, flesh only	5.0	1¼	N	N	N	4g each	0.2	0
Citrus fruit, soft/easy peelers, flesh only, weighed without peel	9.6	2½	6.1	1.9	1.6	60g each	5.8	1½
Citrus fruit, soft/easy peelers, flesh only, weighed with peel	7.5	2	4.8	1.5	1.2	70g each	5.3	1¼
Coconut, flesh only, fresh	3.7	1	3.7	Tr	Tr	100g snack pack	3.7	1
Cranberries	3.4	¾	Tr	1.2	2.2	1g each	0.0	0
Currants	67.8	17	Tr	33.3	34.4	1 heaped tablespoon (25g)	17	4¼
Custard apple, flesh only	14.9	3¾	3.9	5.6	5.4	1 whole small fruit (500g)	74.5	18½
Damsons, flesh and skin, raw, weighed without stones	9.6	2½	1.0	3.4	5.2	15g each	1.4	¼
Damsons, flesh and skin, raw, weighed with stones	8.6	2¼	0.9	3.1	4.7	25g each	2.2	½
Damsons, stewed with sugar, weighed without stones	19.3	4¾	11.1	3.4	4.9	140g	27	6¾
Damsons, stewed without sugar, weighed without stones	8.7	2¼	0.8	3.1	4.8	140g	12.2	3
Dates, dried, flesh and skin, weighed without stone	68.0	17	Tr	32.6	35.4	15g each	10.2	2½
Dates, raw, flesh and skin, weighed without stone	31.3	7¾	Tr	15.1	16.2	25g each	7.8	2
Dried mixed fruit	68.1	17	0.8	31.6	33.3	1 heaped tablespoon (25g)	17.0	4¼
Durian, flesh only	23.2	5¾	N	N	N	½ small fruit (500g)	116.0	29
Elderberries, whole fruit	7.4	1¾	0.3	N	N	1 tablespoon (25g)	1.9	½
Figs, dried, stewed with sugar	34.3	8½	6.7	12.3	15.4	140g	48.0	12
Figs, dried, stewed without sugar	29.4	7¼	0.8	12.7	15.9	140g	41.2	10¼
Figs, ready-to-eat, semi-dried	48.6	12¼	1.5	20.8	26.2	20g each	9.7	2
Figs, whole fruit, dried	52.9	13¼	1.6	22.7	28.6	16g each	8.5	2

Food name	Total sugars (g/100g)	Teaspoons (tsp) sugar/100g	Sucrose (g/100g)	Fructose (g/100g)	Glucose (g/100g)	Average portion size	Grams (g) sugar per average portion	Tsp sugar per average portion
Figs, whole green fruit, raw	9.5	2½	0.3	4.1	5.2	55g each	5.2	1¼
Fruit cocktail, canned in juice, whole contents	11.7	3.0	0.8	5.7	5.2	115g	13.5	3¼
Fruit cocktail, canned in syrup, whole contents	14.8	3¾	1.9	6.4	6.1	115g	16.1	4
Fruit salad, homemade	14.0	3½	6.2	4.6	3.3	140g	19.6	5
Gooseberries, cooking, raw	3.0	¾	Tr	1.6	1.3	6g each	0.2	0
Gooseberries, cooking, stewed with sugar	12.9	3¼	7.8	2.6	2.4	140g	18.1	4½
Gooseberries, cooking, stewed without sugar	2.5	¾	Tr	1.3	1.1	140g	3.5	1
Gooseberries, dessert, canned in syrup, whole contents	18.5	4¾	3.7	7.3	7.5	½ 300g can (150g)	27.8	7
Gooseberries, dessert, raw	9.2	2¼	0.4	4.5	4.3	7g each	0.6	¼
Grapefruit, canned in juice, whole contents	7.3	1¾	0.3	3.4	3.6	120g	8.8	2¼
Grapefruit, canned in syrup, whole contents	15.5	4	1.9	6.9	6.7	120g	18.6	4¾
Grapefruit, flesh only, raw, weighed with peel and pips	4.6	1¼	1.6	1.6	1.4	1 small (250g) 1 medium (340g) 1 large (425g)	11.5 15.6 19.6	2¾ 4 5
Grapefruit, raw, flesh only	6.8	1¾	2.4	2.3	2.1	½ fruit (80g)	5.4	1½
Grapes, average	16.1	4	Tr	8.6	7.5	small bunch (100g)	16.1	4
Grapes, average, weighed with pips	15.8	4	Tr	8.4	7.4	5g each	0.8	¼
Grapes, green	15.2	3¾	Tr	7.9	7.3	5g each	0.8	¼
Grapes, red	17.0	4¼	Tr	9.3	7.7	5g each	0.9	¼
Greengages, raw	9.7	2½	2.7	2.2	4.7	50g each	4.9	1¼
Greengages, raw, weighed with stones	9.2	2¼	2.6	2.1	4.5	55g each	5.1	1¼
Greengages, stewed with sugar, weighed without stones	20.7	5¼	13.0	2.7	4.9	140g	29	7¼
Greengages, stones removed, stewed without sugar	8.7	2¼	2.2	2.1	4.3	140g	12.2	3
Grenadillas, flesh and seeds	7.5	2	2.4	2.2	2.9	85g each	6.4	1½
Guava, canned in syrup, whole contents	15.7	4	3.7	6.5	5.5	1 x 410g can	64.4	16

Food name

Food name	Total sugars (g/100g)	Teaspoons (tsp) sugar/100g	Sucrose (g/100g)	Fructose (g/100g)	Glucose (g/100g)	Average portion size	Grams (g) sugar per average portion	Tsp sugar per average portion
Guava, flesh only, raw	4.9	1¼	0.5	2.3	2.1	100g serving	4.9	1¼
Guava, raw, weighed with skin and pips	4.4	1	0.5	2.1	1.9	1 400g fruit	86.2	21½
Jackfruit, canned, drained	24.8	6¼	13.1	6.2	5.5	½ 567g can (284g)	70.4	17½
Jackfruit, raw	20.6	5¼	10.9	5.1	4.5	200g	41.2	10¼
Jujube, flesh only	19.7	5	N	N	N	15g each	3	¾
Kiwi fruit, flesh and seeds	10.3	2½	1.3	4.3	4.6	60g each	6.2	1½
Kiwi fruit, flesh and seeds, weighed with skin	8.9	2¼	1.1	3.7	4.0	65g each	5.8	1½
Kumquats, canned in syrup, whole contents	35.4	8¾	N	N	N	140g	49.6	12½
Kumquats, whole fruit, raw	9.3	2¼	3.6	3.1	2.6	8g each	0.7	¼
Lemon juice, fresh	1.6	½	0.2	0.9	0.5	juice from ½ lemon (10g)	0.2	0
Lemon juice, fresh, weighed as whole fruit	0.6	¼	0.1	0.3	0.2	1 slice for drinks (20g)	0.1	0
Lemons, flesh only, raw, weighed with peel and pips	1.4	¼	0.3	0.4	0.6	small (100g) large (170g)	1.4 2.4	¼ ½
Lime juice, fresh	1.6	½	0.4	0.6	0.6	juice from ½ lime (5g)	0.1	0
Limes, flesh only, weighed with peel and pips	0.6	¼	0.1	0.2	0.2	30g each	0.2	0
Loganberries, raw	3.4	¾	0.2	1.3	1.9	1 cup (147g)	5	1¼
Loganberries, stewed with sugar	12.5	3¼	9.0	1.5	2.0	115g	14.4	3½
Loganberries, stewed without sugar	2.9	¾	0.2	1.1	1.6	115g	3.3	¾
Longans, canned in syrup, whole contents	16.4	4	N	N	N	1 small can (233g)	38.2	9½
Longans, flesh only, dried	71.5	18	N	N	N	6g each	4.3	1
Loquats, canned in syrup, whole contents	22.2	5	N	N	N	115g	25.5	6¼
Loquats, flesh only, raw	6.3	1½	0.6	3.0	2.7	13g each	0.8	¼
Lychees, canned in syrup, whole contents	17.7	4½	0.6	8.6	8.5	½ can (115g)	20.4	5
Lychees, flesh only, raw, weighed with skin and stone	8.9	1¼	Tr	4.5	4.3	22g each	2	½

Food name	Total sugars (g/100g)	Teaspoons (tsp) sugar/100g	Sucrose (g/100g)	Fructose (g/100g)	Glucose (g/100g)	Average portion size	Grams (g) sugar per average portion	Tsp sugar per average portion
Lychees, raw, flesh only	14.3	3½	Tr	7.3	7.0	15g each	2.1	½
Mammy apple, flesh only	14.4	3½	N	N	N	½ fruit (423g)	60.9	15¼
Mandarin oranges, canned in juice, whole contents	7.7	2	1.8	3.1	2.8	½ 300g can (150g)	11.6	4
Mandarin oranges, canned in syrup, whole contents	13.4	3¼	5.1	4.2	4.1	½ 300g can (150g)	20.1	5
Mangoes, ripe, canned in syrup, whole contents	20.2	5	4.4	8.8	7.0	105g	21.2	5¼
Mango, unripe, green flesh, raw	5.6	1½	0.1	2.0	3.5	1 whole (150g)	8.4	2
Mangoes, ripe, flesh only, raw, weighed with skin and stone	9.4	2	6.9	2.0	0.5	1 whole (200g)	18.8	4¾
Mangoes, ripe, raw, flesh only	13.8	3½	10.1	3.0	0.7	1 slice (40g)	5.5	1½
Mangosteen, flesh only	16.1	4	N	N	N	95g each	15.3	3¾
Matoki (East African Highland Banana), boiled in water	0.6	¼	0.6	Tr	Tr	140g	0.8	¼
Matoki (East African Highland Banana), raw	0.9	¼	0.7	0.1	0.1	1 whole fruit (100g)	0.9	¼
Medlars, flesh only	10.6	2¾	N	N	N	60g each	5.7	1½
Melon, Canteloupe-type, flesh only	4.2	1	0.1	2.2	1.8	1 slice (150g)	6.3	1½
Melon, Galia, flesh only	5.6	1½	2.0	2.0	1.6	1 slice (150g)	8.4	2
Melon, Honeydew, flesh only	4.0	1	1.5	1.5	1.0	1 slice (200g)	8	2
Melon, watermelon, flesh only	7.1	1¾	3.4	2.3	1.3	1 slice (200g)	14.2	3½
Melon, yellow flesh, flesh only	6.8	1¾	2.6	2.5	1.7	1 slice (150g)	10.2	2½
Mulberries, whole fruit, raw	8.1	2	Tr	4.3	3.8	100g	8.1	2
Mulberries, whole fruit, stewed with sugar	16.2	4	8.9	3.9	3.5	140g	22.7	5¾
Mulberries, whole fruit, stewed without sugar	6.9	1¾	Tr	3.7	3.3	140g	9.7	2½
Nectarines, flesh and skin	9.0	2¼	6.3	1.3	1.3	90g each	8.1	2
Nectarines, flesh and skin, weighed with stones	8.0	2	5.6	1.2	1.2	120g	1.2	¼
Oranges, flesh only	8.2	2	4.0	2.2	2.0	1 small (120g) 1 medium (160g) 1 large (210g)	9.8 13.1 17.2	2½ 3¼ 4¼
Oranges, flesh only, weighed with peel	5.8	1½	2.8	1.6	1.4	200g each	11.6	3

Food name	Total sugars (g/100g)	Teaspoons (tsp) sugar/100g	Sucrose (g/100g)	Fructose (g/100g)	Glucose (g/100g)	Average portion size	Grams (g) sugar per average portion	Tsp sugar per average portion
Ortaniques, flesh only	11.7	3	N	N	N	70g each	8.2	2
Papaya, canned in juice, whole contents	17.0	4¼	2.2	7.0	7.8	small (113g) pot	19.2	4¾
Papaya, raw, flesh only	8.8	2¼	3.1	2.8	2.8	1 slice (140g)	12.3	3
Papaya, raw, flesh only, weighed with skin and pips	6.6	1¾	2.3	2.1	2.1	1 whole fruit (454g)	30	7½
Passion fruit, flesh and pips	5.8	1½	1.7	1.9	2.2	15g each	0.9	¼
Passion fruit, flesh and pips, weighed with skin	3.5	½	1.0	1.1	1.3	35g each	1.2	¼
Peaches, canned in juice, whole contents	9.7	2½	3.6	3.7	2.4	120g	11.6	3
Peaches, canned in syrup, whole contents	14.0	3½	6.7	3.6	3.7	120g	16.8	4¼
Peaches, dried	53.0	13¼	37.1	7.9	7.9	20g each	10.6	2¾
Peaches, dried, stewed with sugar	25.7	6½	17.6	4.0	4.0	140g	36	9
Peaches, dried, stewed without sugar	21.7	5½	13.7	3.9	3.9	140g	30.4	7½
Peaches, flesh and skin, raw, weighed with stone	6.8	1¾	4.7	1.0	1.0	150g each	10.2	2½
Peaches, raw, flesh and skin, weighed without stone	7.6	2	5.2	1.1	1.1	1 small (70g) 1 medium (110g) 1 large (150g)	5.3 8.4 11.4	1¼ 2 2¾
Pears, average, flesh and skin, raw, weighed with core and stalk	9.2	2¼	1.0	5.6	2.6	medium Comice pear (150g) medium Conference pear (170g)	13.8 15.6	3½ 4
Pears, average, stewed with sugar	18.8	4¾	10.9	5.4	2.5	140g	26.3	6½
Pears, average, stewed without sugar	9.8	2½	1.0	6.0	2.8	140g	13.7	3½
Pears, canned in juice, whole contents	8.5	2¼	0.6	5.7	2.3	½ a pear (60g) average portion (135g)	5.1 11.5	1¼ 3¾
Pears, canned in syrup, whole contents	13.2	3¼	3.4	6.1	3.4	½ a pear (60g) average portion (135g)	7.9 17.8	2 4½
Pears, dried	52.4	13	3.6	36.8	11.9	½ dried pear (20g)	10.5	2½

Food name	Total sugars (g/100g)	Teaspoons (tsp) sugar/100g	Sucrose (g/100g)	Fructose (g/100g)	Glucose (g/100g)	Average portion size	Grams (g) sugar per average portion	Tsp sugar per average portion
Pears, Nashi, flesh and skin, raw, weighed with core	6.3	1½	Tr	4.4	2.0	140g each	8.8	2¼
Physalis, fruit only	11.1	2¾	N	N	N	6g each	0.7	¼
Pineapple, canned in juice, whole contents	12.2	3	4.2	4.0	4.0	1 ring or 6 chunks (40g)	4.9	1¼
Pineapple, canned in syrup, whole contents	16.5	4¼	5.8	4.8	6.0	1 ring or 6 chunks (40g)	6.6	1¾
Pineapple, dried	67.9	17	37.3	17.0	13.6	100g pack 25g snack pack	67.9 17.0	17 4¼
Pineapple, flesh only, raw, weighed with skin and top	5.3	1¼	2.9	1.3	1.1	1 whole fruit (1000g)	53	13¼
Pineapple, raw, flesh only	10.1	2½	5.5	2.5	2.0	1 large slice (80g)	8.1	2
Plums, average, flesh and skin, stewed with sugar, weighed with stones	17.0	4¼	12.0	1.6	3.4	140g	23.8	6
Plums, average, flesh and skin, stewed without sugar	7.3	1¾	2.1	1.7	3.6	120g	8.8	2¼
Plums, average, flesh and skin, stewed without sugar, weighed with stones	6.9	1¾	2.0	1.6	3.4	140g	9.7	2½
Plums, average, raw, flesh and skin	8.8	2¼	2.5	2.0	4.3	small (30g) medium (55g) large (85g)	2.6 4.8 7.5	¾ 1¼ 1¾
Plums, average, raw, flesh and skin, weighed with stones	8.3	2	2.3	1.9	4.0	1 average (80g)	6.6	1¾
Plums, average, flesh and skin, stewed with sugar, weighed without stones	17.9	4½	12.6	1.7	3.6	120g	21.5	5¼
Plums, canned in syrup, whole contents	15.5	4	2.2	6.2	7.1	⅓ 570g can (190g)	29.4	7¼
Pomegranate, flesh and pips	11.8	3	0.2	5.2	6.4	from 1 whole fruit (156g)	18.4	4½
Pomegranate, flesh and pips, weighed with skin	7.7	2	0.1	3.4	4.2	1 whole fruit (255g)	19.6	5
Pomelo, flesh only	6.8	1¾	2.4	2.3	2.1	165g	11.2	2¾
Pomelo, flesh only, weighed with peel and pips	4.1	1	1.5	1.4	1.3	1 slice of a whole, 1kg, small fruit (100g)	4.1	1

Food name	Total sugars (g/100g)	Teaspoons (tsp) sugar/100g	Sucrose (g/100g)	Fructose (g/100g)	Glucose (g/100g)	Average portion size	Grams (g) sugar per average portion	Tsp sugar per average portion
Prickly pears, flesh and seeds	11.5	3	0.1	5.4	6.0	102g each	11.7	3
Prunes, canned in juice, whole contents	19.7	5	1.1	8.4	10.2	½ 290g can (145g)	28.6	7¼
Prunes, canned in syrup, whole contents	23.0	5¾	6.5	5.5	11.0	½ 290g can (145g)	33.4	8¼
Prunes, flesh and skin	38.4	9½	4.5	13.7	20.2	25g each	9.6	2½
Prunes, flesh and skin, stewed with sugar	25.5	6½	8.4	7.0	10.1	6 pieces (60g)	15.3	3¾
Prunes, flesh and skin, stewed with sugar, weighed with stones	23.5	6	7.7	6.4	9.3	115g	27	6¾
Prunes, flesh and skin, stewed without sugar	19.5	5	2.1	7.1	10.4	6 pieces (60g)	11.7	4
Prunes, flesh and skin, stewed without sugar, weighed with stones	17.8	4½	1.9	6.4	9.4	115g	20.5	5
Prunes, flesh and skin, raw, weighed with stones	32.3	8	3.9	11.8	16.7	30g each	9.7	2½
Prunes, ready-to-eat, semi-dried	34.0	8½	4.1	12.1	17.9	6g each	2	½
Prunes, ready-to-eat, semi-dried, weighed with stones	29.2	7¼	3.4	10.4	15.4	8g each	2.7	¾
Quinces, flesh only	6.3	1½	0.3	3.7	2.3	1 whole medium fruit (450g)	28.4	7
Raisins	69.3	17¼	Tr	34.8	34.5	1 tablespoon (30g)	20.8	5¼
Rambutan, flesh only	16.3	4	10.3	3.1	2.9	40g each	6.5	2½
Raspberries, canned in syrup, whole contents	22.5	5¾	N	N	N	average portion (90g)	20.3	5
Raspberries, raw	4.6	1¼	0.2	2.4	1.9	4g each	0.2	0
						average portion, 15 raspberries (60g)	2.8	¾
Raspberries, stewed with sugar	15.0	3¾	10.1	2.7	2.2	120g	18	4½
Raspberries, stewed without sugar	4.4	1	0.2	2.3	1.8	120g	5.3	1¼
Redcurrants, raw	4.4	1	0.1	2.6	1.7	½ 150g pack (75g)	3.3	¾
Redcurrants, stewed with sugar	13.3	3¼	8.9	2.5	1.8	120g	16	4

Food name	Total sugars (g/100g)	Teaspoons (tsp) sugar/100g	Sucrose (g/100g)	Fructose (g/100g)	Glucose (g/100g)	Average portion size	Grams (g) sugar per average portion	Tsp sugar per average portion
Redcurrants, stewed without sugar	3.8	1	0.1	2.2	1.5	120g	4.6	1¼
Rhubarb, canned in syrup, whole contents	7.6	2	2.1	2.6	2.9	½ 539g can (270g)	20.5	5
Rhubarb, stems only, raw	0.8	¼	0.1	0.4	0.4	1 stalk (40g)	0.3	0
Rhubarb, stems only, stewed with sugar	11.5	3	9.1	1.2	1.2	140g	16.1	4
Rhubarb, stems only, stewed without sugar	0.7	¼	0.1	0.3	0.3	140g	1.0	¼
Sapodilla, flesh only	14.7	3¾	2.7	5.3	6.7	1 whole fruit (150g)	22.1	5½
Sharon fruit, flesh only	18.6	4¾	Tr	9.3	9.3	1 whole fruit (110g)	20.5	5
Star fruit	7.1	1¾	0.8	3.2	3.1	1 whole medium fruit (100g)	7.1	1¾
Strawberries, canned in syrup, whole contents	16.9	4¼	7.3	4.9	4.7	90g	15.2	3¾
Strawberries, raw	6.1	1½	Tr	3.1	3.0	12g each average portion (100g)	0.7 / 6.1	¼ / 1½
Sugar apple (custard apple), flesh only	14.9	3¾	3.9	5.6	5.4	1 whole small fruit (500g)	74.5	18½
Sultanas	69.4	17¼	Tr	34.6	34.8	1 tablespoon (30g)	20.8	5¼
Tamarillos, flesh and seeds	4.7	1¼	2.4	1.2	1.1	1 whole fruit (100g)	4.7	1¼
Whitecurrants, raw	5.6	1½	0.8	2.3	2.4	½ 150g pack (75g)	19.7	5
Whitecurrants, stewed with sugar	14.2	3½	9.5	2.3	2.4	120g	17.0	4¼
Whitecurrants, stewed without sugar	4.8	1¼	0.6	2.0	2.1	120g	5.8	1½

Grains and cereals

Food name	Total sugars (g/100g)	Teaspoons (tsp) sugar/100g	Sucrose (g/100g)	Fructose (g/100g)	Glucose (g/100g)	Average portion size	Grams (g) sugar per average portion	Tsp sugar per average portion
Baby cereals, rice-based	6.3	1½	3.3	0.1	0.5	1 tablespoon (5g)	0.3	0
Baby cereals, various cereal-based	23.5	6	7.6	1.8	3.2	1 tablespoon (5g)	1.2	¼
Baby cereals, wheat-based	9.7	2½	2.9	0.2	0.3	1 tablespoon (5g)	0.5	¼
Barley, pearl, boiled	Tr	0	Tr	Tr	Tr	1 tablespoon (20g)	Tr	0
Barley, pearl, raw	Tr	0	Tr	Tr	Tr	1 tablespoon dried, after boiling (60g)	Tr	0
Bran, wheat	2.3	½	2.3	Tr	Tr	1 tablespoon (7g)	0.2	0
Breakfast cereal, bran flakes, fortified	21.0	5¼	15.9	2.6	2.0	1 tablespoon (8g)	1.7	½
Breakfast cereal, bran type cereal, fortified	20.0	5	17.5	0.7	0.7	1 tablespoon (7g)	1.4	¼
Breakfast cereal, cornflakes, crunchy / honey nut coated, fortified	37.4	9¼	33.1	1.6	2.7	1 tablespoon (8g)	3	¾
Breakfast cereal, cornflakes, fortified	7.3	1¾	4.1	1.5	1.7	1 tablespoon (6g)	0.4	0
Breakfast cereal, cornflakes, frosted, fortified	38.3	9½	36.2	1.0	1.1	1 tablespoon (8g)	3.1	¾
Breakfast cereal, cornflakes, unfortified	3.0	¾	1.7	0.6	0.7	1 tablespoon (6g)	0.2	0
Breakfast cereal, crunchy clusters type, without nuts, unfortified	25.3	6¼	16.6	3.8	3.6	1 tablespoon (20g)	5.1	1¼
Breakfast cereal, crunchy/crispy muesli type cereal, with nuts, unfortified	23.1	5¾	20.2	1.6	1.4	1 average portion (30g)	6.9	1¾
Breakfast cereal, fruit and fibre type, fortified	26.2	6½	8.4	9.4	8.4	1 tablespoon (8g)	2.1	½
Breakfast cereal, Grapenuts	12.1	3	0.0	4.3	1.0	1 tablespoon (7g)	0.8	¼
Breakfast cereal, honey loops and hoops, including Honey and Nut Cheerios, fortified	34.7	8¾	31.0	1.6	1.4	1 tablespoon (5g)	1.7	½
Breakfast cereal, instant hot oat, plain, raw, fortified	0.5	¼	0.2	Tr	Tr	1 tablespoon (7g)	0	0
Breakfast cereal, malted flake, fortified	17.2	¼	14.9	0.5	0.3	1 tablespoon (8g)	1.4	¼

Food name	Total sugars (g/100g)	Teaspoons (tsp) sugar/100g	Sucrose (g/100g)	Fructose (g/100g)	Glucose (g/100g)	Average portion size	Grams (g) sugar per average portion	Tsp sugar per average portion
Breakfast cereal, malted wheat, fortified	20.3	4	18.9	0.4	0.3	1 tablespoon (8g)	1.6	½
Breakfast cereal, multigrain hoops, fortified	22.4	5½	N	N	N	1 tablespoon (5g)	1.1	¼
Breakfast cereal, oat, instant, flavoured, unfortified, made up with semi-skimmed milk	7.8	2	4.1	Tr	Tr	small portion made with ⅙ pint milk (130g)	10.1	2½
						medium portion made with ¼ pint milk (180g)	14.0	3½
						large portion made with ⅓ pint milk (225g)	17.6	4½
Breakfast cereal, oat, instant, plain, fortified, cooked, made up with semi-skimmed milk	4.2	1	Tr	Tr	Tr	small portion made with ⅙ pint milk (130g)	5.5	1½
						medium portion made with ¼ pint milk (180g)	7.6	2
						large portion made with ⅓ pint milk (225g)	9.4	2¼
Breakfast cereal, puffed wheat, honey coated, fortified	36.8	9¼	N	N	N	1 tablespoon (6g)	2.2	½
Breakfast cereal, puffed wheat, unfortified	0.2	0	Tr	0.2	Tr	1 tablespoon (3g)	0	0
Breakfast cereal, rice, chocolate flavoured, fortified	37.7	9½	36.9	0.4	0.5	1 tablespoon (4g)	1.5	½
Breakfast cereal, rice, toasted/crisp, fortified	12.4	3	11.6	0.5	0.3	1 tablespoon (4g)	0.5	¼
Breakfast cereal, Ricicles, Kellogg's	39.1	9¾	38.8	0.2	0.1	1 tablespoon (4g)	1.6	½
Breakfast cereal, shredded wheat type with fruit, unfortified	18.7	4¾	8.0	6.0	4.7	average portion (45g)	8.4	2
Breakfast cereal, shredded wheat type, unfortified	0.6	¼	0.6	Tr	Tr	22g each	0.1	0
Breakfast cereal, Shredded Wheat, honey nut, Nestle	19.6	5	18.1	0.9	0.6	average portion (45g)	8.8	2¼
Breakfast cereal, Start	31.3	7¾	23.1	1.5	2.0	1 tablespoon (6g)	1.9	½
Breakfast cereal, sultana bran, fortified	29.2	7¼	7.1	11.5	10.6	1 tablespoon (8g)	2.3	½

Food name	Total sugars (g/100g)	Teaspoons (tsp) sugar/100g	Sucrose (g/100g)	Fructose (g/100g)	Glucose (g/100g)	Average portion size	Grams (g) sugar per average portion	Tsp sugar per average portion
Breakfast cereal, wheat and multigrain, chocolate flavoured, fortified	30.5	7¾	30.0	0.1	0.2	1 tablespoon (7g)	2.1	½
Breakfast cereal, wheat biscuits, Weetabix type, fortified	3.9	1	1.9	0.9	0.7	20g each	0.8	¼
Breakfast cereal, wheat biscuit with fruit, fortified	24.4	6	18.7	3.6	2.2	1 tablespoon (7g)	1.7	½
Buckwheat, groats	0.4	0	Tr	Tr	Tr	100g	0.4	0
Cereal bars, with fruit and/or nuts, no chocolate, unfortified	34.3	8½	9.5	9.0	9.9	1 whole bar (42g)	14.4	3½
Cereal bars, with fruit and/or nuts, with chocolate, unfortified	40.7	10¼	25.9	6.5	6.4	1 whole bar (29g)	11.8	3
Couscous, plain, cooked	1.0	¼	0.2	Tr	Tr	small portion (150g)	1.5	½
Couscous, plain, raw	2.3	½	0.8	Tr	Tr	1 tablespoon (33g)	0.8	¼
Muesli, luxury	25.1	6¼	Tr	12.7	12.4	1 tablespoon (15g)	3.8	1
Muesli, Swiss style, no added sugar or salt, unfortified	13.0	3¼	Tr	5.2	4.6	1 tablespoon (15g)	2	½
Muesli, Swiss style, unfortified	21.3	5¼	7.4	5.0	4.9	1 tablespoon (15g)	3.2	¾
Polenta, hydrated, raw	Tr	0	Tr	Tr	Tr	½ 500g packet (250g)	Tr	0
Porridge oats, unfortified	0.3	0	0.3	Tr	Tr	1 tablespoon (7g)	0	0
Porridge oats, unfortified, cooked, made up with semi-skimmed milk	4.1	1	Tr	Tr	Tr	small portion (110g)	4.5	1¼
						medium portion (160g)	6.6	1¾
						large portion (210g)	8.6	2¼
Porridge, made with milk and water	2.5	¾	0.0	Tr	Tr	small portion (110g)	2.8	¾
						medium portion (160g)	4.0	1
						large portion (210g)	5.3	1¼

Food name	Total sugars (g/100g)	Teaspoons (tsp) sugar/100g	Sucrose (g/100g)	Fructose (g/100g)	Glucose (g/100g)	Average portion size	Grams (g) sugar per average portion	Tsp sugar per average portion
Porridge, made with water	Tr	0	Tr	Tr	Tr	small portion (110g)	Tr	0
						medium portion (160g)	Tr	0
						large portion (210g)	Tr	0
Porridge, made with whole milk	4.8	1¼	0.0	Tr	Tr	small portion (110g)	5.3	1¼
						medium portion (160g)	7.7	2
						large portion (210g)	10.1	2½
Quinoa, raw	6.1	1½	2.8	0.6	2.7	¼ 300g packet (75g)	4.6	1¼
Sago, raw	Tr	0	0.0	0.0	Tr	50g	Tr	0
Semolina, raw	0.6	¼	0.4	Tr	Tr	¼ 500g packet (125g)	0.8	¼
Wheat, bulgur, raw	1.1	¼	1.0	Tr	Tr	¼ 500g packet (125g)	1.4	¼
Wheatgerm	16.0	4	14.8	0.5	0.7	1 tablespoon (5g)	0.8	¼

Herbs and spices

Although dried herbs and spice might
contain quite a lot of sugar, remember
that you will only ever be using a
tiny amount in cooking.

Food name	Total sugars (g/100g)	Teaspoons (tsp) sugar/100g	Sucrose (g/100g)	Fructose (g/100g)	Glucose (g/100g)	Average portion size	Grams (g) sugar per average portion	Tsp sugar per average portion
Chilli powder	7.2	1¾	0.8	4.3	2.1	1 teaspoon (3g)	0.2	0
Chives, fresh	1.9	½	Tr	1.0	0.9	¼ of a 25g fresh pack (6.25g)	0.1	0
Cinnamon, ground	2.2	½	Tr	1.1	1.0	1 teaspoon (3g)	0	0
Coriander leaves, fresh	0.9	¼	Tr	0.4	0.5	¼ of a 31g fresh pack (17.75g)	0.2	0
Cumin seeds	2.3	½	N	N	N	1 teaspoon (2g)	0	0
Curry paste	7.0	1¾	N	N	N	45g	3.1	¾
Dill, dried	37.6	9½	14.1	9.4	14.1	1 teaspoon (1g)	0.4	0
Dill, fresh	0.8	¼	0.3	0.2	0.3	1 tablespoon (3g)	0	0
Garlic powder	4.2	1	1.5	1.6	1.1	1 teaspoon (3g)	0.1	0
Garlic puree	16.9	4¼	3.7	6.8	6.4	1 teaspoon (3g)	0.5	¼
Garlic, raw	1.6	½	0.6	0.6	0.4	1 clove (13g)	0.2	0
Ginger, fresh	1.7	½	0.0	0.9	0.8	5 slices (11g)	0.2	0
Ginger, ground	19.8	5	0.0	10.2	9.6	1 teaspoon (3g)	0.6	¼
Horseradish, raw	7.3	1¾	6.5	0.1	0.7	1 teaspoon (5g)	0.4	0
Nutmeg, ground	28.5	7¼	N	N	N	1 teaspoon (3g)	0.9	¼
Oregano, dried, ground	4.1	1	0.9	1.1	1.9	1 teaspoon (1g)	0	0
Oregano, fresh	0.8	¼	0.2	0.2	0.4	1 heaped tablespoon (3g)	0	0
Paprika	10.3	2½	0.8	6.7	2.6	1 teaspoon (3g)	0.3	0
Parsley, dried	12.4	3	N	4.8	7.5	1 level teaspoon (1g)	0.1	0
Parsley, fresh	2.3	½	Tr	0.9	1.4	1 large sprig (1g)	0	0
Pepper, black	0.6	¼	Tr	0.2	0.2	1 level teaspoon (2g)	0	0
Peppers, capsicum, chilli, green, raw	0.7	¼	0.1	0.2	0.4	45g each	0.3	0
Peppers, capsicum, chilli, red, raw	4.2	1	Tr	2.3	1.9	45g each	1.9	½
Saffron	42.4	10½	N	N	N	1 teaspoon (3g)	1.3	¼
Salt	0.0	0	0.0	0.0	0.0	1 level teaspoon (5g)	0	0
Tamarind pulp, flesh only	64.5	16¼	N	N	N	1 teaspoon (5g)	3.2	¾
Thyme, dried, ground	1.7	½	N	N	N	1 teaspoon (1g)	0	0
Thyme, fresh	0.6	0	N	N	N	1 4 inch sprig (1g)	0	0

Meat and meat products

Fresh meat and poultry have no sugar, but meat products might have some sugar that is added during food processing.

Food name	Total sugars (g/100g)	Teaspoons (tsp) sugar/100g	Sucrose (g/100g)	Fructose (g/100g)	Glucose (g/100g)	Average portion size	Grams (g) sugar per average portion	Tsp sugar per average portion
Bacon loin steaks, lean, grilled	1.1	¼	N	N	N	170g each	1.9	½
Bacon rashers	0.0	0	0.0	0.0	0.0	1 rasher streaky bacon (20g)	0.0	0
						1 rasher back bacon (25g)	0.0	0
Bacon rashers, sweetcure	1.6	½	0.0	0.0	0.0	1 rasher streaky bacon (20g)	0.3	0
						1 rasher back bacon (25g)	0.4	0
Bacon fat	0.0	0	0.0	0.0	0.0	1oz (28g)	0.0	0
Beef, braising steak	0.0	0	0.0	0.0	0.0	medium portion (140g)	0.0	0
						large portion (210g)	0.0	0
Beef, brisket	0.0	0	0.0	0.0	0.0	medium portion (90g)	0.0	0
						large portion (150g)	0.0	0
Beef, fillet steak	0.0	0	0.0	0.0	0.0	5oz, fried (108g) grilled (105g)	0.0	0
						8oz, fried (172g) grilled (168g)	0.0	0
Beef, rump steak	0.0	0	0.0	0.0	0.0	5oz, fried (103g) grilled (102g)	0.0	0
						8oz, fried (166g) grilled (163g)	0.0	0
Beef, silverside	0.0	0	0.0	0.0	0.0	5oz minute steak, fried (80g)	0.0	0
						grilled (78g)	0.0	0
Beef, sirloin steak	0.0	0	0.0	0.0	0.0	T-bone steak: 8oz, fried (169g) grilled (166g)	0.0	0
						12oz, fried (253g) grilled (248g)	0.0	0
Beef, topside	0.0	0	0.0	0.0	0.0	thin slice roast beef (28g)	0.0	0
Black pudding, dry-fried	0.2	0	0.1	Tr	0.1	1 slice (30g)	0.1	0
Burger, beef, 62–85%, beef, grilled	2.1	½	N	N	N	56g raw, 40g when cooked	0.8	¼
						quarter pounder, 90g when cooked	1.9	½

Food name	Total sugars (g/100g)	Teaspoons (tsp) sugar/100g	Sucrose (g/100g)	Fructose (g/100g)	Glucose (g/100g)	Average portion size	Grams (g) sugar per average portion	Tsp sugar per average portion
Burger, beef, 98–99% beef, fried or grilled	0.1	0	0.0	0.0	0.1	quarterpounder, 78g when cooked	0.0	0
Burger, beef, fried or grilled, homemade	0.8	¼	0.3	0.2	0.3	80% beef, 56g raw, 36g when cooked	0.3	0
						100% beef, 56g raw, 34g when cooked	0.3	0
Chital, raw (Imported frozen from Bangladesh)	0.0	0	0.0	0.0	0.0	1oz (28g)	0.0	0
Chorizo	1.1	¼	Tr	0.0	0.0	1 small slice, 5 cm diameter (5g)	0.0	0
						1 large slice, 11cm diameter (12g)	0.1	0
Corned beef, canned	1.0	¼	0.9	0.0	0.1	1 thick slice (50g)	0.5	¼
						1 small can (198g)	2.0	½
Frankfurter	1.1	¼	Tr	Tr	0.2	small (23g)	0.3	0
						large (47g)	0.5	¼
Haggis, boiled	Tr	0	Tr	Tr	Tr	1 thin slice (14g)	0.0.	0
Ham	1.0	¼	N	N	N	1 thin slice (14g)	0.1	0
Ham, gammon joint	0.0	0	0.0	0.0	0.0	average slice (23g)	0.0	0
Ham, gammon rashers, grilled	0.0	0	0.0	0.0	0.0	170g each	0.0	0
Hare	0.0	0	0.0	0.0	0.0	120g	0.0	0
Heart	0.0	0	0.0	0.0	0.0	1 whole cooked, lamb's (200g)	0.0	0
Kidney	0.0	0	0.0	0.0	0.0	1 whole lamb's fried (35g)	0.0	0
						1 tablespoon cooked (40g)		
Kofta, beef, homemade	0.8	¼	0.3	0.2	0.3	90g	0.7	¼
Kofta, lamb, coated with breadcrumbs, homemade	0.9	¼	N	N	N	95g	0.9	¼
Lamb, cutlets	0.0	0	0.0	0.0	0.0	with bone (98g)	0.0	0
						edible portion (50g)	0.0	0

Food name	Total sugars (g/100g)	Teaspoons (tsp) sugar/100g	Sucrose (g/100g)	Fructose (g/100g)	Glucose (g/100g)	Average portion size	Grams (g) sugar per average portion	Tsp sugar per average portion
Lamb, chops, fried or grilled	0.0	0	0.0	0.0		braising chop, with bone (120g)	0.0	0
						edible portion (70g)	0.0	0
Lamb, roast joint (breast or leg)	0.0	0	0.0	0.0	0.0	small portion (50g)	0.0	0
						medium portion (90g)	0.0	0
						large portion (150g)	0.0	0
						average slice (30g)	0.0	0
Lamb, steaks	0.0	0	0.0	0.0	0.0	chump chop, with bone (120g)	0.0	0
						edible portion (70g)	0.0	0
Lamb, mince	0.0	0	0.0	0.0	0.0	1oz (28g)	0.0	0
Lamb, mince, stewed with onions	0.6	¼	0.2	0.2	0.2	260g	1.6	½
Lamb, shoulder, diced, kebabs, grilled, lean and fat	0.0	0	0.0	0.0	0.0	85g	0.0	0
Liver and bacon, fried, homemade	0.0	0	Tr	0.0	0.0	142g	0.0	0
Liver sausage	1.0	¼	0.0	0.0	1.0	1 slice (14g)	0.1	0
Liver, fried	0.0	0	0.0	0.0	0.0	100g	0.0	0
Luncheon meat, canned	Tr	0	Tr	Tr	Tr	average slice (14g)	0.0	0
Meat spread	0.2	0	0.1	0.0	0.1	15g	0.0	0
Oxtail, stewed	0.0	0	0.0	0.0	0.0	260g	0.0	0
Pate, liver	0.4	0	0.0	0.0	0.4	1 tablespoon (35g)	0.1	0
Pate, meat, reduced fat	1.3	¼	0.1	0.0	1.1	1 tablespoon (35g)	0.5	¼
Polony	Tr	0	Tr	Tr	Tr	30g	0.0	0
Pork chops in mustard and cream, homemade	1.1	¼	0.1	0.3	0.3	85g	0.9	¼
Pork chops in mustard and cream, homemade, weighed with bone	1.0	¼	0.1	0.2	0.3	165g	1.7	½
Pork, belly joint/slices	0.0	0	0.0	0.0	0.0	110g	0.0	0

Food name	Total sugars (g/100g)	Teaspoons (tsp) sugar/100g	Sucrose (g/100g)	Fructose (g/100g)	Glucose (g/100g)	Average portion size	Grams (g) sugar per average portion	Tsp sugar per average portion
Pork, chump chops/ steaks, fried	0.0	0	0.0	0.0	0.0	135g	0.0	0
Pork, crackling, cooked	0.0	0	0.0	0.0	0.0	35g	0.0	0
Pork, diced, casseroled	0.0	0	0.0	0.0	0.0	75g	0.0	0
Pork, diced, kebabs	0.0	0	0.0	0.0	0.0	75g	0.0	0
Pork, fillet slices, grilled	0.0	0	0.0	0.0	0.0	75g	0.0	0
Pork, fillet strips, stir-fried in oil	0.0	0	0.0	0.0	0.0	75g	0.0	0
Pork, roast joint	0.0	0	0.0	0.0	0.0	1 average slice (40g)	0.0	0
Pork, loin chops	0.0	0	0.0	0.0	0.0	170g	0.0	0
Pork, loin steaks, fried	0.0	0	0.0	0.0	0.0	120g	0.0	0
Pork, mince	0.0	0	0.0	0.0	0.0	1oz (28g)	0.0	0
Pork, spare rib chops	0.0	0	0.0	0.0	0.0	with bone (220g) without bone (140g)	0.0 0.0	0 0
Pork, spare rib joint	0.0	0	0.0	0.0	0.0	150g	0.0	0
Pork, spare rib slices/ steaks	0.0	0	0.0	0.0	0.0	75g	0.0	0
Pork, spare ribs, 'barbecue style', homemade, weighed with bone	1.1	¼	0.1	0.3	0.3	220g	2.4	½
Pork, spare ribs, 'barbecue style', meat only, retail, reheated, weighed with bone	1.0	¼	0.1	0.2	0.3	140g	1.4	¼
Pork, spare ribs, 'barbecue style', meat only, retail, reheated	0.0	0	0.0	0.0	0.0	140g	0.0	0
Pork, spare ribs, in black bean sauce, meat and sauce only, homemade	0.0	0	0.0	0.0	0.0	220g	0.0	0
Pork, spare ribs, in black bean sauce, meat and sauce only, homemade, weighed with bone	0.0	0	0.0	0.0	0.0	140g	0.0	0
Pork, steaks	0.0	0	0.0	0.0	0.0	135g	0.0	0
Rabbit, stewed	0.0	0	0.0	0.0	0.0	1 whole rabbit (850g)	0.0	0

Food name	Total sugars (g/100g)	Teaspoons (tsp) sugar/100g	Sucrose (g/100g)	Fructose (g/100g)	Glucose (g/100g)	Average portion size	Grams (g) sugar per average portion	Tsp sugar per average portion
Salami	0.5	¼	0.0	0.0	0.1	1 small slice, 5cm diameter (5g)	0.0	0
						1 large slice, diameter 11cm (12g)	0.1	0
						1 snack salami, pepperoni (25g)	0.1	0
Sausages, beef, fried in oil	2.6	¾	0.8	0.2	0.4	40g each	1.0	¼
Sausages, beef, grilled	2.4	½	0.7	0.2	0.4	40g each	1.0	¼
Sausages, beef, raw	2.6	¾	0.4	0.1	0.5	57g each	1.5	½
Sausages, pork, chilled, fried or grilled	1.6	½	0.2	Tr	0.4	40g each	0.6	¼
Sausages, pork, raw	2.8	¾	Tr	Tr	1.1	57g each	1.6	½
Sausages, pork, reduced fat, fried	2.6	¾	0.1	0.0	0.9	40g each	1.0	¼
Sausages, pork, reduced fat, grilled	3.4	¾	0.1	0.0	1.2	40g each	1.4	¼
Sausages, pork, reduced fat, raw	3.5	1	0.1	0.0	1.2	57g each	2.0	½
Sausages, premium, fried	1.0	¼	0.1	0.0	0.8	50g each	0.5	¼
Sausages, premium, grilled	0.9	¼	0.1	0.0	0.7	50g each	0.5	¼
Sausages, premium, raw	1.5	½	0.2	0.0	1.2	67g	1.0	¼
Tongue, pickled	0.0	0	0.0	0.0	0.0	1 slice (25g)	0.0	0
Tongue, stewed	0.0	0	0.0	0.0	0.0	1 slice (25g)	0.0	0
Tongue slices	Tr	0	Tr	Tr	Tr	1 slice (25g)	0.0	0
Tripe and onions, stewed, homemade	4.8	1¼	0.8	0.6	0.8	150g	7.2	1¾
Veal, escalope	0.0	0	0.0	0.0	0.0	150g	0.0	0
Veal, mince	0.0	0	0.0	0.0	0.0	1oz (28g)	0.0	0
Venison, roast	0.0	0	0.0	0.0	0.0	120g	0.0	0
White pudding	Tr	0	Tr	Tr	Tr	1 slice (30g)	0.0	0
Wiener schnitzel, homemade	0.7	¼	0.1	0.1	0.0	150g	1.1	¼

Milk and dairy products

Food name	Total sugars (g/100g)	Teaspoons (tsp) sugar/100g	Sucrose (g/100g)	Fructose (g/100g)	Glucose (g/100g)	Average portion size	Grams (g) sugar per average portion	Tsp sugar per average portion
Buttermilk	5.0	1¼	0.0	0.0	0.0	1 tablespoon (15g)	0.8	¼
Buttermilk powder	51.0	12¾	0.0	0.0	0.0	1 teaspoon (3g)	1.5	½
Cheese spread, flavoured	4.4	1	0.0	0.0	0.0	triangle (17g)	0.8	¼
Cheese spread, plain	6.5	1 ¾	0.0	0.0	0.0	triangle (17g)	1.1	¼
Cheese spread, plain, reduced fat	7.3	1¾	0.0	0.0	0.0	triangle (17g)	1.2	¼
Cheese, Brie, with outer rind	Tr	0	0.0	0.0	0.0	average portion (30g)	0.0	0
Cheese, Caerphilly	0.1	0	0.0	0.0	0.0	average portion (30g)	0.0	0
Cheese, Camembert	Tr	0	0.0	0.0	0.0	40g	0.0	0
Cheese, Cheddar type, '30% less fat'	0.1	0	0.0	0.0	0.0	grated, 1 tablespoon (10g)	0.0	0
						matchbox size piece (30g)	0.0	0
						in sandwich, average (45g)	0.0	0
Cheese, Cheddar type, half fat	Tr	0	0.0	0.0	0.0	grated, 1 tablespoon (10g)	0.0	0
						matchbox size piece (30g)	0.0	0
						in sandwich, average (45g)	0.0	0
Cheese, Cheddar, English	0.1	0	0.0	0.0	0.0	grated, 1 tablespoon (10g)	0.0	0
						matchbox size piece (30g)	0.0	0
						in sandwich, average (45g)	0.0	0
Cheese, cottage, plain	3.1	¾	0.0	0.0	0.0	1 tablespoon (40g)	1.2	¼
Cheese, cottage, plain, reduced fat	3.3	¾	0.0	0.0	0.0	1 tablespoon (40g)	1.3	¼
Cheese, cottage, plain, with additions	2.6	¾	0.0	0.0	0.6	1 tablespoon (40g)	1.0	¼
Cheese, Danish blue	Tr	0	0.0	0.0	0.0	average portion (30g)	0.0	0
Cheese, dairy free hard cheese alternative (e.g. soya)	Tr	0	0.0	0.0	0.0	average portion (30g)	0.0	0

Food name	Total sugars (g/100g)	Teaspoons (tsp) sugar/100g	Sucrose (g/100g)	Fructose (g/100g)	Glucose (g/100g)	Average portion size	Grams (g) sugar per average portion	Tsp sugar per average portion
Cheese, Derby	0.1	0	0.0	0.0	0.0	average portion (30g)	0.0	0
Cheese, Dolcelatte, rind removed	Tr	0	0.0	0.0	0.0	average portion (30g)	0.0	0
Cheese, Double Gloucester	0.1	0	0.0	0.0	0.0	average portion (30g)	0.0	0
Cheese, Edam	Tr	0	0.0	0.0	0.0	average portion (30g)	0.0	0
Cheese, Emmental	Tr	0	0.0	0.0	0.0	average portion (30g)	0.0	0
Cheese, Feta	1.5	½	0.0	0.0	0.0	average portion (30g)	0.5	¼
Cheese, goats milk, full fat, soft, white rind	1.0	¼	0.0	0.0	0.0	average portion (30g)	0.3	0
Cheese, Gouda	Tr	0	0.0	0.0	0.0	average portion (30g)	0.0	0
Cheese, Gruyere	Tr	0	0.0	0.0	0.0	average portion (30g)	0.0	0
Cheese, Halloumi	1.7	½	0.0	0.0	0.0	average portion (30g)	0.5	¼
Cheese, hard, average	0.1	0	0.0	0.0	0.0	average portion (30g)	0.0	0
Cheese, Lancashire	0.1	0	0.0	0.0	0.0	average portion (30g)	0.0	0
Cheese, Mascarpone	4.3	1	0.0	0.0	0.0	average portion (30g)	1.3	¼
Cheese, Mozzarella, fresh	Tr	0	0.0	0.0	0.0	average portion (30g)	0.0	0
Cheese, Paneer	0.9	¼	0.0	0.0	0.0	average portion (30g)	0.3	0
Cheese, Parmesan, fresh	0.9	¼	0.0	0.0	0.0	average portion (30g)	0.3	0
Cheese, Port Salut, St Paulin type	Tr	0	0.0	0.0	0.0	average portion (30g)	0.0	0
Cheese, processed, plain	5.0	1¼	0.0	0.0	0.0	1 slice (20g)	1.0	¼
Cheese, processed, slices, reduced fat	7.6	2	0.0	0.0	0.0	1 slice (20g) 1 triangle (17g)	1.5 1.3	½ ¼
Cheese, processed, smoked	0.2	0	0.0	0.0	0.0	average portion (30g)	0.1	0

Food name	Total sugars (g/100g)	Teaspoons (tsp) sugar/100g	Sucrose (g/100g)	Fructose (g/100g)	Glucose (g/100g)	Average portion size	Grams (g) sugar per average portion	Tsp sugar per average portion
Cheese, Quark	4.0	1	0.0	0.0	0.0	1 heaped tablespoon (55g)	2.2	½
Cheese, Red Leicester	0.1	0	0.0	0.0	0.0	average portion (30g)	0.0	0
Cheese, Red Windsor	Tr	0	0.0	0.0	0.0	average portion (30g)	0.0	0
Cheese, Ricotta	2.0	½	0.0	0.0	0.0	average portion (30g)	0.6	¼
Cheese, Roquefort	Tr	0	0.0	0.0	0.0	average portion (30g)	0.0	0
Cheese, Sage Derby	0.1	0	0.0	0.0	0.0	average portion (30g)	0.0	0
Cheese, spreadable, full fat, soft, white	3.0	¾	0.0	0.0	0.0	individual pot (17g)	0.5	¼
						in sandwich, average (30g)	0.9	¼
Cheese, spreadable, medium fat, soft, white	3.5	1	0.0	0.0	0.0	individual pot (17g)	0.6	¼
						in sandwich, average (30g)	1.0	¼
Cheese, spreadable, soft white, low fat	5.0	1¼	0.0	0.0	0.0	individual pot (17g)	0.9	¼
						in sandwich, average (30g)	1.5	½
Cheese, Stilton, blue	0.1	0	0.0	0.0	0.0	35g	0.0	0
Cheese, Stilton, white	0.1	0	0.0	0.0	0.0	35g	0.0	0
Cheese, Wensleydale	0.1	0	0.0	0.0	0.0	average portion (30g)	0.0	0
Cheese, White Cheshire	0.1	0	0.0	0.0	0.0	average portion (30g)	0.0	0
Cheese, white, average	0.1	0	0.0	0.0	0.0	individually wrapped e.g. mini Babybel (18g)	0.0	0
Coffeemate, whitener powder	9.4	2¼	0.0	0.0	5.0	1 teaspoon (3g)	0.3	0
						1 heaped tablespoon (4.5g)	0.4	0
Cream substitute, double	3.6	1	0.0	0.0	0.0	1 tablespoon (15g)	0.5	0
Cream substitute, single	4.0	1	0.0	0.0	0.0	1 tablespoon (15g)	0.6	¼

Food name	Total sugars (g/100g)	Teaspoons (tsp) sugar/100g	Sucrose (g/100g)	Fructose (g/100g)	Glucose (g/100g)	Average portion size	Grams (g) sugar per average portion	Tsp sugar per average portion
Cream substitute, whipping (e.g. Elmlea)	3.3	¾	0.0	0.0	0.0	1 tablespoon (15g)	0.5	¼
						1 tablespoon whipped (30g)	1.0	¼
Cream, dairy, extra thick (24% fat)	3.4	¾	0.0	0.0	0.0	1 tablespoon (25g)	0.9	¼
Cream, dairy, UHT, canned spray, 85% cream (squirty)	7.2	1¾	3.9	0.0	0.0	1 tablespoon (10g)	0.7	¼
Cream, dairy, UHT, half fat, canned spray (squirty)	7.4	1¾	3.8	0.0	0.0	1 tablespoon (10g)	0.7	¼
Cream, fresh, clotted	2.3	½	0.0	0.0	0.0	average serving (38g)	0.9	¼
Cream, fresh, double, including Jersey cream	1.7	½	0.0	0.0	0.0	1 tablespoon (15g)	0.3	0
Cream, fresh, single	2.2	½	0.0	0.0	0.0	1 tablespoon (15g)	0.3	0
Cream, fresh, whipping	2.7	¾	0.0	0.0	0.0	1 tablespoon (15g)	0.4	0
Cream, half, fresh	4.3	1	0.0	0.0	0.0	1 tablespoon (15g)	0.6	¼
Cream, half, UHT	4.3	1	0.0	0.0	0.0	1 tablespoon (15g)	0.6	¼
Creme fraiche, full fat	2.1	½	0.0	0.0	0.0	1 tablespoon (40g)	0.8	¼
Creme fraiche, half fat	3.0	¾	0.0	0.0	0.0	1 tablespoon (40g)	1.2	¼
Cream, single, UHT	4.0	1	0.0	0.0	0.0	1 tablespoon (15g)	0.6	¼
Cream, soured, fresh	3.8	1	0.0	0.0	0.0	1 tablespoon (25g)	1.0	¼
Cream, sterilised, canned	3.7	1	0.0	0.0	0.0	1 tablespoon (15g)	0.6	¼
Cream, whipping, UHT	3.1	¾	0.0	0.0	0.0	1 tablespoon whipped (30g)	0.9	¼
Fromage frais, fruit, children's, fortified	11.8	0	N	N	N	small children's pot (60g)	7.1	1¾
Fromage frais, virtually fat free, fruit	4.9	1¼	0.2	0.9	0.7	1 tablespoon (45g)	2.2	½
Fromage frais, virtually fat free, natural	4.4	1	0.0	0.0	0.2	1 tablespoon (45g)	2.0	½

Food name	Total sugars (g/100g)	Teaspoons (tsp) sugar/100g	Sucrose (g/100g)	Fructose (g/100g)	Glucose (g/100g)	Average portion size	Grams (g) sugar per average portion	Tsp sugar per average portion
Milk, 1% fat, pasteurised	4.8	1¼	0.0	0.0	0.0	1 tablespoon (15g)	0.7	¼
						small glass (200g)	9.6	2½
Milk, Channel Islands, whole, pasteurised	4.3	1	0.0	0.0	0.0	1 tablespoon (15g)	0.6	¼
						small glass (200g)	8.6	2¼
Milk, Channel islands, whole, summer	4.1	1	0.0	0.0	0.0	1 tablespoon (15g)	0.6	¼
						small glass (200g)	8.2	2
Milk, Channel islands, whole, winter	4.4	1	0.0	0.0	0.0	1 tablespoon (15g)	0.7	¼
						small glass (200g)	8.8	2¼
Milk, condensed, skimmed, sweetened	60.0	15	46.7	0.0	0.0	1 can (405g)	243.0	60¾
Milk, condensed, whole, sweetened	55.5	14	43.2	0.0	0.0	1 can (397g)	220.3	60
Milk, evaporated, light	10.3	2½	0.0	0.0	0.0	1 small can (170g)	17.5	4½
Milk, evaporated, whole	12.7	3 ¼	0.0	0.0	0.0	1 small can (170g)	21.6	5½
Milk, flavoured, pasteurised, chocolate	11.0	2 ¾	2.8	1.7	Tr	200ml carton (227g)	25.0	6¼
Milk, flavoured, pasteurised, strawberry, banana	8.9	2 ¼	3.9	Tr	Tr	200ml carton (227g)	20.2	5
Milk, goats, pasteurised	4.4	1	0.0	0.0	0.0	1 tablespoon (15g)	0.7	¼
						small glass (200g)	8.8	2¼
Milk, semi-skimmed, pasteurised, average	4.7	1 ¼	0.0	0.0	0.0	1 tablespoon (15g)	0.7	¼
						small glass (200g)	9.4	2¼
Milk, semi-skimmed, pasteurised, summer and autumn	4.5	1 ¼	0.0	0.0	0.0	1 tablespoon (15g)	0.7	¼
						small glass (200g)	9.0	2¼

Food name	Total sugars (g/100g)	Teaspoons (tsp) sugar/100g	Sucrose (g/100g)	Fructose (g/100g)	Glucose (g/100g)	Average portion size	Grams (g) sugar per average portion	Tsp sugar per average portion
Milk, semi-skimmed, pasteurised, winter and spring	4.9	1 ¼	0.0	0.0	0.0	1 tablespoon (15g)	0.7	¼
						small glass (200g)	9.8	2½
Milk, semi-skimmed, UHT	4.9	1 ¼	0.0	0.0	0.0	1 tablespoon (15g)	0.7	¼
						small glass (200g)	9.8	2½
Milk, sheeps, raw	5.1	1 ¼	0.0	0.0	0.0	1 tablespoon (15g)	3.7	1
						small glass (200g)	10.2	2½
Milk, skimmed, dried, fortified	52.9	13 ¼	0.0	0.0	0.0	1 teaspoon (3g)	1.6	½
Milk, skimmed, dried, fortified, with vegetable fat	42.6	10 ¾	0.0	0.0	0.0	1 teaspoon (3g)	1.3	¼
Milk, skimmed, pasteurised, average	4.8	1¼	0.0	0.0	0.0	1 tablespoon (15g)	0.7	¼
						small glass (200g)	9.6	2½
Milk, skimmed, pasteurised, summer	4.4	1	0.0	0.0	0.0	1 tablespoon (15g)	0.7	¼
						small glass (200g)	8.8	2¼
Milk, skimmed, pasteurised, winter	4.2	1	0.0	0.0	0.0	1 tablespoon (15g)	0.6	¼
						small glass (200g)	8.4	2¼
Milk, skimmed, sterilised	5.4	1¼	0.0	0.0	0.0	1 tablespoon (15g)	0.8	¼
						small glass (200g)	10.8	2½
Milk, skimmed, UHT	4.9	1¼	0.0	0.0	0.0	1 tablespoon (15g)	0.7	¼
						small glass (200g)	9.8	2½
Milk, soya, non-dairy alternative to milk, sweetened, fortified	2.2	½	0.7	1.2	0.3	1 tablespoon (15g)	0.3	0
						small glass (200g)	4.4	1
Milk, soya, non-dairy alternative to milk, unsweetened, fortified	0.2	0	0.2	0.0	0.0	1 tablespoon (15g)	0.0	0
						small glass (200g)	0.4	0

Food name	Total sugars (g/100g)	Teaspoons (tsp) sugar/100g	Sucrose (g/100g)	Fructose (g/100g)	Glucose (g/100g)	Average portion size	Grams (g) sugar per average portion	Tsp sugar per average portion
Milk, soya, non-dairy alternative to milk, unsweetened, unfortified	0.2	0	0.2	0.0	0.0	1 tablespoon (15g)	0.0	0
						small glass (200g)	0.4	0
Milk, whole, dried	39.4	9¾	0.0	0.0	0.0	1 teaspoon (3g)	1.2	¼
Milk, whole, pasteurised, average	4.6	1¼	0.0	0.0	0.0	1 tablespoon (15g)	0.7	¼
						small glass (200g)	9.2	2¼
Milk, whole, pasteurised, summer and autumn	4.1	1	0.0	0.0	0.0	1 tablespoon (15g)	0.6	¼/
						small glass (200g)	8.2	2
Milk, whole, pasteurised, winter and spring	5.0	1¼	0.0	0.0	0.0	1 tablespoon (15g)	0.8	¼
						small glass (200g)	10.0	2½
Milk, whole, sterilised	4.5	1¼	0.0	0.0	0.0	1 tablespoon (15g)	0.7	¼
						small glass (200g)	9.0	2¼
Milk, whole, UHT	4.8	1¼	0.0	0.0	0.0	1 tablespoon (15g)	0.7	¼
						small glass (200g)	9.6	2½
Tip Top dessert topping	7.1	1¾	0.3	0.0	0.0	3 tablespoons (50g)	3.6	1
Yogurt, drinking, UHT	13.1	3¼	6.0	1.1	1.3	200ml pot (212g)	27.8	7
Yogurt, goats, whole milk	3.9	1	0.0	0.0	0.0	142g pot	5.5	1½
Yogurt, Greek style, fruit	10.5	2¾	3.8	1.0	Tr	1 tablespoon (45g)	4.7	1¼
Yogurt, Greek style, plain (full fat)	4.5	1¼	Tr	Tr	0.1	1 tablespoon (45g)	2.0	½
Yogurt, low fat, fruit	12.7	3¼	6.1	1.0	Tr	1 tablespoon (40g)	5.1	1¼
Yogurt, low fat, hazelnut	14.9	3¾	7.9	0.8	Tr	1 tablespoon (40g)	6.0	1½
Yogurt, low fat, plain	7.5	2	0.0	0.0	0.0	1 tablespoon (40g)	3.0	¾
Yogurt, low fat, toffee	16.8	4¼	10.4	0.5	Tr	1 tablespoon (40g)	6.7	1¾
Yogurt powder	54.4	13½	0.0	0.0	0.0	1oz (28g)	15.2	3¾

Food name	Total sugars (g/100g)	Teaspoons (tsp) sugar/100g	Sucrose (g/100g)	Fructose (g/100g)	Glucose (g/100g)	Average portion size	Grams (g) sugar per average portion	Tsp sugar per average portion
Yogurt, soya, non-dairy alternative to yogurt, fruit, fortified	10.7	2¾	6.7	1.7	2.3	120g pot	12.8	3¼
Yogurt, virtually fat free/diet, fruit (including bio varieties)	9.4	2¼	2.1	0.5	1.3	1 tablespoon (40g)	3.8	1
Yogurt, virtually fat free/diet, plain (including bio varieties)	7.9	2	0.1	Tr	1.6	1 tablespoon (40g)	3.2	¾
Yogurt, virtually fat free/diet, twin pot, fruit	6.8	1¾	Tr	1.3	0.7	1 tablespoon (40g)	2.7	¾
Yogurt, whole milk, fruit (including bio varieties)	16.6	4¼	6.2	2.2	3.3	125g pot	20.1	5
Yogurt, whole milk, infant, fruit flavour	10.4	2½	4.5	1.5	Tr	large children's yoghurt pot (100g)	10.4	2½
Yogurt, whole milk, plain	7.8	2	0.0	0.0	0.0	150g pot	11.7	3
Yogurt, whole milk, twin pot, not fruit (with biscuit pieces and chocolate-coated cereal pieces)	18.2	0	N	N	N	135g pot	24.6	6¼
Yogurt, whole milk, twin pot, thick and creamy with fruit	15.6	4	6.9	2.2	2.3	150g pot	23.4	5¾

Non-alcoholic drinks and beverages

A cup is equivalent to 250ml when filled
to the rim. However, very few people
fill their cups that way, and so we have
calculated the sugar content per 240ml.

For cup sizes, we have estimated a
cup size of 150ml when the cup is filled
to about 1.5 cm (about half an inch)
below the rim.

Food name	Total sugars (g/100g)	Teaspoons (tsp) sugar/100g	Sucrose (g/100g)	Fructose (g/100g)	Glucose (g/100g)	Average portion size	Grams (g) sugar per average portion	Tsp sugar per average portion
Apple juice, clear, ambient and chilled	9.7	2	1.8	5.5	2.4	small glass (160g) tall tumbler (300g)	15.5 29.1	4 7¼
Baby fruit juice, fortified with vitamin C	8.0	2	0.9	4.9	2.2	125 ml carton (130g) 250ml carton (260g)	10.4 20.8	2½ 5¼
Barley water, diluted (diluted 1:4)	4.3	1	N	N	N	small glass 160ml (176g) tall tumbler 300ml (330g)	7.6 14.2	2 3½
Barley water, undiluted	21.5	5½	N	N	N	average measure (50g)	10.8	2¾
Blackcurrant squash, diluted	7.2	1¾	4.8	1.0	1.2	diluted 1:4 (250g)	18	4½
Blackcurrant squash, undiluted	54.2	8½	36.3	7.8	8.8	average measure (50g)	27.1	6¾
Carrot juice	5.7	1½	3.5	0.9	1.3	small glass 160ml (163g) tall tumbler 300ml (306g)	9.3 17.4	2¼ 4¼
Cocoa powder, made up with semi-skimmed milk	6.5	1¾	2.0	0.0	0.0	1 mug 240 ml (252g)	16.4	4
Cocoa powder, made up with skimmed milk	6.5	1¾	2.0	0.0	0.0	1 mug 240 ml (254g)	16.5	4¼
Cocoa powder, made up with whole milk	6.3	1½	2.0	0.0	0.0	1 mug 240 ml (252g)	15.9	4
Coffee and chicory essence (e.g. Camp coffee), undiluted	53.8	8½	47.5	3.4	2.9	1 level tablespoon (25g)	13.5	4
Coffee and chicory essence (e.g. Camp coffee), with water	2.3	½	2.0	0.1	0.1	1 average cup (190g) 1 average mug (260g)	4.4 6.0	1 1½
Coffee, cappuccino, latte (unsweetened)	2.4	½	0.0	0.0	0.0	1 sachet (13g)	0.3	0
Coffee, infusion, black	0	0	0	0	0	1 average cup (190g) 1 average mug (260g)	0.0 0.0	0 0
Coffee, infusion, average, with semi-skimmed milk	0.7	¼	0.0	0.0	0.0	1 average cup (190g) 1 average mug (260g)	1.3 1.8	¼ ½
Coffee, infusion, average, with single cream	0.3	0	0.0	0.0	0.0	1 average cup (190g) 1 average mug (260g)	0.6 0.8	¼ ¼
Coffee, infusion, average, with whole milk	0.5	¼	0.0	0.0	0.0	1 average cup (190g) 1 average mug (260g)	1.0 1.3	¼ ¼
Coffee, instant, made up with water	0.0	0	0.0	0.0	0.0	1 average cup (190g) 1 average mug (260g)	0.0 0.0	0 0

Food name	Total sugars (g/100g)	Teaspoons (tsp) sugar/100g	Sucrose (g/100g)	Fructose (g/100g)	Glucose (g/100g)	Average portion size	Grams (g) sugar per average portion	Tsp sugar per average portion
Coffee, instant, made up with water and semi-skimmed milk	0.7	¼	0.0	0.0	0.0	1 average cup (190g)	1.3	¼
						1 average mug (260g)	1.8	½
Coffee, instant, made up with water and whole milk	0.5	¼	0.0	0.0	0.0	1 average cup (190g)	1.0	¼
						1 average mug (260g)	1.3	¼
Coffee, powder, instant	0.0	0	0.0	0.0	0.0	1 heaped teaspoon (2g)	0.0	0
Cola	10.9	2¾	4.0	3.4	3.5	500ml bottle (520g)	56.7	14¼
						330ml can (343g)	37.4	9¼
Cola, diet	Tr	0	Tr	Tr	Tr	500ml bottle (520g)	Tr	0
						330ml can (343g)	Tr	0
Cranberry fruit juice drink	12.1	3	N	N	N	small glass 160ml (165g)	20.0	5
						tall tumbler 300ml (309g)	37.4	9¼
						200ml carton (206g)	25.0	6¼
Drinking chocolate powder, made up with semi-skimmed milk	10.7	2¾	6.4	0.0	0.0	1 mug 240ml (252g)	27.0	6¾
Drinking chocolate powder, made up with skimmed milk	10.8	2¾	6.4	0.0	0.0	1 mug 240ml (254g)	27.4	6¾
Drinking chocolate powder, made up with whole milk	10.6	2¾	6.4	0.0	0.0	1 mug 240ml (252g)	26.7	6¾
Drinking chocolate, powder	77.7	19½	77.7	0.0	0.0	1 average sachet (11g)	8.5	2¼
Drinking chocolate, powder, reduced fat	82.1	20½	81.2	0.9	Tr	1 average sachet (11g)	9.0	2¼
Energy drink, carbonated	11.1	2¾	N	N	N	500ml bottle (520g)	57.7	14
						330ml can (343g)	38.1	½
Fruit juice drink, carbonated, no added sugar, ready to drink	0.6	¼	0.3	0.2	0.1	small glass 160ml (166g)	1.0	¼
						tall tumbler 300 ml (312g)	1.9	½
						200ml carton (208g)	1.2	¼
Fruit juice drink, carbonated, ready to drink, with sugar	7.2	1¾	N	N	N	small glass 160ml (166g)	12.0	3
						tall tumbler 300ml (312g)	22.5	5¾
						200ml carton (208g)	15.0	3¾
						150ml mini Britvic can (156g)	11.2	2¾
Fruit juice drink, no added sugar, ready to drink	0.9	¼	0.3	0.3	0.3	small glass 160ml (162g)	1.5	½
						tall tumbler 300ml (303g)	2.7	¾
						200ml carton (202g)	1.8	½
Fruit juice drink/squash, diluted (diluted 1:4)	1.8	½	0.2	0.7	0.7	small glass 160ml (174g)	3.1	¾
						tall tumbler 300ml (327g)	5.9	1½

Food name	Total sugars (g/100g)	Teaspoons (tsp) sugar/100g	Sucrose (g/100g)	Fructose (g/100g)	Glucose (g/100g)	Average portion size	Grams (g) sugar per average portion	Tsp sugar per average portion
Fruit juice drink/squash, no sugar added, diluted (diluted 1:4)	0.3	0	0.0	0.1	0.1	small glass 160ml (162g)	0.5	¼
						tall tumbler 300ml (303g)	0.9	¼
Fruit juice drink/squash, no sugar added, undiluted	1.4	¼	0.2	0.7	0.5	average measure (50g)	0.7	¼
Fruit juice drink/squash, ready to drink	9.8	2½	3.4	3.7	2.7	small glass 160ml (165g)	16.2	4
						tall tumbler 300ml (309g)	30.3	7½
						200ml carton (206g)	20.2	5
Fruit juice drink/squash, undiluted	8.9	2¼	1.2	3.7	3.7	average measure (50g)	4.5	1¼
Fruit juice, mixed	10.3	2½	N	N	N	small glass 160ml (163g)	16.8	4¼
						tall tumbler 300ml (306g)	31.5	7¾
						200ml carton (204g)	21.0	4¼
						150ml mini Britvic can (153g)	15.8	4
Ginger ale, dry	3.9	1	0.5	1.6	1.7	500 ml bottle (520g)	20.3	5
						330ml can or bottle (343g)	13.4	3¼
						small 150ml can (156g)	6.1	1½
Grape juice, unsweetened	16.0	4	Tr	8.5	7.5	small glass 160ml (163g)	26.1	6½
						tall tumbler 300ml (306g)	49.0	11¾
Grapefruit juice, unsweetened	8.3	2	2.0	3.3	3.0	small glass 160ml (163g)	13.5	3
						tall tumbler 300ml (306g)	25.4	6¼
High juice drink, diluted	8.5	2¼	2.0	3.2	3.3	small glass 160ml (166g)	14.1	3½
						tall tumbler 300ml (312g)	26.5	6¾
High juice drink, no added sugar, undiluted	4.6	1¼	2.2	1.3	1.1	average measure (50g)	2.3	½
High juice drink, undiluted	42.6	10¾	9.8	16.2	16.6	average measure (50g)	21.3	5¼
Horlicks powder, made up with semi-skimmed milk	8.5	2¼	N	N	N	1 mug 240ml (250g)	21.3	5¼
Horlicks powder, made up with skimmed milk	8.5	2¼	N	N	N	1 mug 240ml (250g)	21.3	5¼
Horlicks powder, made up with whole milk	8.4	2	N	N	N	1 mug 240ml (250g)	21.0	5¼
Horlicks, powder	38.9	9¾	N	N	N	1 sachet (23g)	8.9	2¼
Instant drinks powder, chocolate, low calorie	33.6	8½	Tr	Tr	0.7	1 small sachet (e.g. Cadbury's Highlights) (11g)	3.7	1
Instant drinks powder, malted, unfortified	54.8	13¾	10.7	0.0	3.7	1 sachet (23g)	12.6	3¼

Food name	Total sugars (g/100g)	Teaspoons (tsp) sugar/100g	Sucrose (g/100g)	Fructose (g/100g)	Glucose (g/100g)	Average portion size	Grams (g) sugar per average portion	Tsp sugar per average portion
Lassi, sweetened	11.9	3	2.3	0.1	0.1	small glass 160ml (170g)	20.2	5
						tall tumbler 300ml (318g)	37.8	9½
Lemonade	5.8	1½	2.8	1.4	1.5	small glass (163g)	9.5	2½
						tall tumbler (306g)	17.7	4½
						200ml carton (204g)	11.8	3
						150ml mini Britvic can (153g)	8.9	2¼
Lemonade, homemade	16.7	4¼	16.7	0.1	Tr	small glass 160ml (163g)	27.2	6¾
						tall tumbler 300ml (306g)	51.1	12¾
Lime juice cordial, diluted	6.0	1½	1.2	2.2	2.3	½ pint (45g cordial)	2.7	¾
						1 pint (90g cordial)	5.4	1¼
Lime juice cordial, undiluted	29.8	7½	5.9	11.0	11.5	½ pint (45g)	13.4	3¼
						1 pint (90g)	26.8	6¾
Lucozade	11.1	2¾	N	N	N	500ml bottle (520g)	57.7	14½
Mango juice, canned	9.6	2½	7.0	2.1	0.5	small glass 160ml (165g)	15.8	4
						tall tumbler 300ml (309g)	29.7	7½
						200ml (206g) carton	19.7	4
Milk drink, fermented, with probiotics	12.3	3	N	N	N	1 mini bottle (100g)	12.3	3
Milk shake, powder	98.3	24½	95.2	0.0	0.1	1 rounded teaspoon (5g)	4.9	1¼
Milk shake, powder, made up with semi-skimmed milk	11.2	2¾	6.6	0.0	0.0	small glass 160ml (170g)	19.0	4
						tall tumbler 300ml (318g)	35.6	¾
Milk shake, powder, made up with skimmed milk	11.3	2¾	6.6	0.0	0.0	small glass 160ml (170g)	19.2	4
						tall tumbler 300ml (318g)	35.9	¾
Milk shake, powder, made up with whole milk	11.1	2¾	6.6	0.0	0.0	small glass 160ml (170g)	18.9	4¾
						tall tumbler 300ml (318g)	35.3	8¾
Milkshake syrup, concentrated	35.5	9	10.1	12.2	13.2	1 level tablespoon (25g)	8.9	2¼
Milkshake syrup, concentrated, made up with semi-skimmed milk	9.3	1¼	1.4	1.7	1.8	small glass 160ml (170g)	15.8	4
						tall tumbler 300ml (318g)	29.6	7½
Milkshake syrup, concentrated, made up with whole milk	9.0	1¼	1.4	1.7	1.8	small glass 160ml (170g)	15.3	3¾
						tall tumbler 300ml (318g)	28.6	7¼
Orange juice, ambient, UHT	8.5	2¼	4.1	2.4	2.0	small glass 160ml (163g)	13.4	3¼
						tall tumbler (306g)	26.0	6½
						200ml carton (204g)	17.3	4¼
						standard 330ml can (337g)	28.6	7¼
						150ml mini Britvic can (153g)	13.0	3¼

Food name	Total sugars (g/100g)	Teaspoons (tsp) sugar/100g	Sucrose (g/100g)	Fructose (g/100g)	Glucose (g/100g)	Average portion size	Grams (g) sugar per average portion	Tsp sugar per average portion
Orange juice, chilled	8.6	2¼	4.2	2.4	2.0	small glass (163g) tall tumbler (306g)	14.0 26.3	3½ 7½
Orange juice, freshly squeezed	8.1	2	4.0	2.2	2.0	small glass (163g) tall tumbler (306g)	13.2 24.8	3¼ 6¼
Orange juice, freshly squeezed, weighed as whole fruit	3.7	1	1.8	1.0	0.9	small glass (163g) tall tumbler (306g)	6.0 11.3	1½ 2¾
Ovaltine powder, made up with semi-skimmed milk	9.5	2½	N	N	N	240ml mug (252g)	23.9	6
Ovaltine powder, made up with skimmed milk	9.6	2½	N	N	N	240ml mug (252g)	24.2	6
Ovaltine powder, made up with whole milk	9.4	2½	N	N	N	240ml mug (252g)	23.7	6
Ovaltine, powder	48.3	12	N	N	N	1 sachet (25g)	12.1	3
Passion fruit juice	10.7	2¾	3.1	3.5	4.1	small glass (163g) tall tumbler (306g)	17.4 32.7	4¼ 8¼
Pineapple juice, unsweetened	10.5	2¾	4.7	2.9	2.9	small glass 160ml (163g) tall tumbler 300ml (306g) 200ml carton (204g) 150ml mini bottle (153g)	17.1 32.1 21.4 16.1	4¼ 8 5¼ 4
Pomegranate juice drink	11.6	3	0.2	5.1	6.3	small glass 160ml (165g) tall tumbler 300ml (309g)	19.1 35.8	4¾ 9
Prune juice	14.4	3½	Tr	4.4	10.0	small glass 160ml (163g)	23.5	6
Root beer	10.6	2¾	N	N	N	375ml bottle (382g)	40.5	10 ¼
Smoothies (Retail, chilled, yellow and red fruit smoothies. Not made with milk.)	11.6	3	N	N	N	small glass 160ml (171g) tall tumbler 300ml (321g) 180ml carton (193g)	19.8 37.2 22.4	5 9¼ 5½
Soda, club	0.0	0	0.0	0.0	0.0	330ml can (337g) 150ml can (153g)	0.0	0
Sunny Delight	9.4	1¼	N	N	N	small glass 160ml (165g) tall tumbler 300ml (309g) 200ml carton (206g)	15.5 29.0 19.4	4 7¼ 4¾
Tea, black, infusion	Tr	0	0.0	0.0	0.0	1 average cup (190g) 1 average mug (260g)	Tr Tr	0 0
Tea, Chinese, leaves, infusion	Tr	0	0.0	0.0	0.0	1 average cup (190g) 1 average mug (260g)	Tr Tr	0 0
Tea, green, infusion	Tr	0	0.0	0.0	0.0	1 average cup (190g) 1 average mug (260g)	Tr Tr	0 0

Food name	Total sugars (g/100g)	Teaspoons (tsp) sugar/100g	Sucrose (g/100g)	Fructose (g/100g)	Glucose (g/100g)	Average portion size	Grams (g) sugar per average portion	Tsp sugar per average portion
Tea, herbal, infusion	0.0	0	0.0	0.0	0.0	1 average cup (190g)	0.0	0
						1 average mug (260g)	0.0	0
Tea, infusion, with semi-skimmed milk	0.7	¼	0.0	0.0	0.0	1 average cup (190g)	1.3	¼
						1 average mug (260g)	1.8	½
Tea, infusion, with whole milk	0.5	¼	0.0	0.0	0.0	1 average cup (190g)	1.0	¼
						1 average mug (260g)	1.3	¼
Tea, lemon, instant powder	81.7	20½	0.0	0.0	81.7	1 teaspoon (2g)	1.6	½
Tea, lemon, instant powder, with water	2.1	½	0.0	0.0	2.1	1 mug 240ml (6g powder)	0.1	0
Tomato juice	3.0	¾	Tr	1.6	1.4	small glass 160ml (166g)	5.0	1¼
						tall tumbler 300ml (312g)	9.4	2¼
						200ml carton (208g)	6.2	1½
						160ml pub bottle (166g)	5.0	1¼
						150ml mini Britvic can (156g)	4.7	1¼
Tonic water	5.9	1½	N	N	N	small 150ml can (153g)	9.0	2¼
Water	0.0	0	0.0	0.0	0.0	large 500ml bottle (500g)	0.0	0
						standard 300ml bottle (300g)	0.0	0

Nuts and seeds

Food name	Total sugars (g/100g)	Teaspoons (tsp) sugar/100g	Sucrose (g/100g)	Fructose (g/100g)	Glucose (g/100g)	Average portion size	Grams (g) sugar per average portion	Tsp sugar per average portion
Almonds, toasted	4.3	1	4.3	Tr	Tr	6 nuts (13g)	0.6	¼
Almonds, weighed with shells	1.5	½	1.5	Tr	Tr	1 nut (1.2g)	0.0	0
Barcelona nuts, kernel only	3.4	¾	3.4	0.0	0.0	5 nuts (6.5g)	0.2	0
Barcelona nuts, kernel only, weighed with shells	2.1	½	2.1	0.0	0.0	1 whole small nut (3g)	0.0	0
Brazil nuts, kernel only	2.4	½	2.4	0.0	0.0	3 nuts (10g)	0.2	0
Brazil nuts, kernel only, weighed with shells	1.1	¼	1.1	0.0	0.0	1 nut (5g)	0.0	0
Cashew nuts, kernel only, plain	4.6	1¼	4.6	0.0	0.0	10 nuts (10g)	0.5	¼
Cashew nuts, kernel only, roasted and salted	5.6	1½	5.6	0.0	0.0	10 nuts (10g)	0.6	¼
Chestnuts, dried	13.2	3¼	13.2	Tr	Tr	1 tablespoon (6g)	0.8	¼
Chestnuts, kernel only, raw	7.0	1¾	7.0	Tr	Tr	5 nuts (50g)	3.5	1
Chestnuts, kernel only, raw, weighed with shells	5.8	1½	5.8	Tr	Tr	1 nut (11g)	0.6	¼
Hazelnuts, kernel only	4.0	1	3.7	0.1	0.2	10 nuts (10g)	0.4	0
Hazelnuts, kernel only, weighed with shells	1.5	½	1.4	Tr	0.1	1 nut (21g)	0.3	0
Macadamia nuts, salted	4.0	1	3.8	0.1	0.1	6 nuts (10g)	0.4	0
Nuts and raisins, mixed	28.8	7¼	3.1	12.9	12.8	small bag (50g)	14.4	3½
Nuts, mixed	5.6	1½	5.6	0.0	0.0	½ 200g bag (50g)	2.8	¾
Peanuts and raisins	34.0	8½	3.5	15.3	15.2	1 handful (40g)	13.6	3½
Peanuts, dry roasted	3.8	1	3.8	0.0	0.0	10 nuts (13g)	0.5	¼
Peanuts, kernel only, plain, unsalted	6.2	1½	6.2	0.0	0.0	10 nuts (13g)	0.8	¼
Peanuts, kernel only, plain, weighed with shells	4.3	1	4.3	0.0	0.0	2g each	0.1	0
Peanuts, raisins and chocolate chips	42.0	10½	14.1	12.9	12.8	¼ 200g bag (50g)	21.0	5¼
Peanuts, roasted and salted	3.8	1	3.8	0.0	0.0	10 nuts (13g)	0.5	¼
Pecan nuts, kernel only	4.3	1	3.7	0.3	0.3	1 nut (6g)	0.3	0
Pecan nuts, kernel only, weighed with shells	2.1	½	1.8	0.1	0.1	1 nut (14g)	0.3	0
Pine nuts, kernel only	3.9	1	3.7	0.1	0.1	1 tablespoon (8.5g)	0.3	0

Food name	Total sugars (g/100g)	Teaspoons (tsp) sugar/100g	Sucrose (g/100g)	Fructose (g/100g)	Glucose (g/100g)	Average portion size	Grams (g) sugar per average portion	Tsp sugar per average portion
Pistachio nuts, kernel only, roasted and salted	5.7	1½	5.7	Tr	Tr	10 nuts (10g)	0.6	¼
Pistachio nuts, kernel only, roasted and salted, weighed with shells	3.2	¾	3.2	Tr	Tr	2g per nut	0.1	0
Pumpkin seeds	1.1	¼	1.1	0.0	0.0	1 tablespoon (16g)	0.2	0
Sesame seeds	0.4	0	0.2	0.1	0.1	1 tablespoon (12g)	0	0
Sunflower seeds	1.7	½	1.7	0.0	0.0	1 tablespoon (16g)	0.3	0
Sunflower seeds, toasted	1.8	½	1.8	0.0	0.0	1 tablespoon (16g)	0.3	0
Walnuts, kernel only	2.6	¾	2.2	0.2	0.2	6 halves (20g)	0.5	¼
Walnuts, kernel only, weighed with shells	1.1	¼	0.9	0.1	0.1	1 walnut (5.3g)	0.1	0

Potatoes and potato dishes

Food name	Total sugars (g/100g)	Teaspoons (tsp) sugar/100g	Sucrose (g/100g)	Fructose (g/100g)	Glucose (g/100g)	Average portion size	Grams (g) sugar per average portion	Tsp sugar per average portion
Potato chips, crinkle cut, frozen, fried	0.9	¼	0.5	0.2	0.2	small portion (100g) medium portion (165g) large portion (240g)	0.9 1.5 2.2	¼ ½ ½
Potato chips, fine cut, frozen, fried	0.6	¼	0.2	0.2	0.2	small portion (100g) medium portion (165g) large portion (240g)	0.6 1.0 1.4	¼ ¼ ¼
Potato chips, homemade, fried	1.5	½	Tr	0.7	0.8	1 chip (10g)	0.2	0
Potato chips, microwave, cooked	0.6	¼	0.3	0.1	0.2	small portion (100g) medium portion (165g) large portion (240g)	0.6 1.0 1.4	¼ ¼ ¼
Potato chips, oven ready, no batter, baked	1.0	¼	0.4	0.3	0.4	1 chip (10g)	0.1	0
Potato chips, oven ready, with batter, baked	0.4	0	0.3	Tr	0.1	small portion (100g) medium portion (165g) large portion (240g)	0.4 0.7 1.0	0 ¼ ¼
Potato chips, straight cut, frozen, fried in blended oil	0.9	¼	0.5	0.2	0.2	small portion (100g) medium portion (165g) large portion (240g)	0.9 1.5 2.2	¼ ½ ½
Potato chips, straight cut, frozen, fried in corn oil	0.3	0	0.3	Tr	Tr	small portion (100g) medium portion (165g) large portion (240g)	0.3 0.5 0.7	0 ¼ ¼
Potato chips, straight cut, frozen, fried in dripping	0.6	¼	0.2	0.2	0.2	small portion (100g) medium portion (165g) large portion (240g)	0.6 1.0 1.4	¼ ¼ ¼
Potato chips, thick cut, frozen, fried in oil	0.6	¼	0.2	0.2	0.2	small portion (100g) medium portion (165g) large portion (240g)	0.6 1.0 1.4	¼ ¼ ¼
Potato croquettes, fried	0.5	¼	0.1	0.3	0.2	1 fried (90g) 1 grilled (80g)	0.5 0.4	¼ 0
Potato fritters, battered, baked	0.3	0	0.2	Tr	0.1	120g each	0.4	0
Potatoes, new, canned, re-heated, drained	0.7	¼	0.5	0.1	0.1	1 whole (300g) can	2.1	½
Potato powder, instant, made up with semi-skimmed milk	1.5	½	Tr	0.1	0.1	1 tablespoon (45g) 1 scoop (60g) 1 forkful (30g)	0.7 0.9 0.5	¼ ¼ ¼
Potato powder, instant, made up with skimmed milk	1.5	½	Tr	0.1	0.1	1 tablespoon (45g) 1 scoop (60g) 1 forkful (30g)	0.7 0.9 0.6	¼ ¼ ¼

Food name	Total sugars (g/100g)	Teaspoons (tsp) sugar/100g	Sucrose (g/100g)	Fructose (g/100g)	Glucose (g/100g)	Average portion size	Grams (g) sugar per average portion	Tsp sugar per average portion
Potato powder, instant, made up with water	0.7	¼	Tr	0.1	0.1	1 tablespoon (45g)	0.3	0
						1 scoop (60g)	0.4	0
						1 forkful (30g)	0.2	0
Potato powder, instant, made up with whole milk	2.0	½	Tr	0.1	0.1	1 tablespoon (45g)	0.9	¼
						1 scoop (60g)	1.2	¼
						1 forkful (30g)	0.6	¼
Potato powder, instant, raw	4.1	1	Tr	0.5	0.5	1 whole small packet (88g)	3.6	1
						½ large (176g) packet (88g)	3.6	1
Potato products, shaped, frozen, baked (including waffles, smiley faces and letters)	0.4	0	0.2	Tr	0.2	1 fried smiley face (9g)	0.0	0
						1 grilled smiley face (6g)	0.0	0
						1 average portion smiley faces (90g)	0.4	0
						1 grilled potato waffle (45g)	0.2	0
Potato wedges, retail, cooked	0.8	¼	0.3	0.2	0.2	average portion (150g)	1.2	¼
Potatoes, duchesse	0.8	¼	0.2	0.3	0.3	30g each	0.2	0
Potatoes, new and salad, boiled in water, flesh and skin	1.1	¼	0.2	0.4	0.5	40g each	0.4	0
Potatoes, new and salad, flesh only, raw	1.3	¼	0.7	0.3	0.3	50g each	0.7	¼
Potatoes, new, frozen, 'roast' in oil	1.0	¼	0.3	0.3	0.4	1 small potato (50g)	0.5	¼
						1 medium potato (85g)	0.9	¼
						1 large potato (130g)	1.3	¼
						average portion (200g)	2.0	½
Potatoes, old, baked, flesh and skin	1.4	¼	0.3	0.5	0.6	small (100g)	1.4	¼
						medium (180g)	2.5	¾
						large (220g)	3.1	¾
Potatoes, old, baked, flesh only	0.7	¼	0.4	0.1	0.2	small (88g)	0.6	¼
						medium (160g)	1.1	¼
						large (195g)	1.4	¼
Potatoes, old, boiled in water, flesh only	0.8	¼	0.2	0.3	0.3	60g each	0.5	¼
Potatoes, old, mashed with butter	1.0	¼	0.2	0.3	0.3	1 tablespoon (45g)	0.5	¼
						1 scoop (60g)	0.6	¼
						1 forkful (30g)	0.3	0
Potatoes, old, mashed with reduced fat spread	1.0	¼	0.2	0.3	0.3	1 tablespoon (45g)	0.5	¼
						1 scoop (60g)	0.6	¼
						1 forkful (30g)	0.3	0
Potatoes, old, microwaved, flesh and skin	2.1	½	0.4	0.8	0.9	125g each	2.6	¾

Food name	Total sugars (g/100g)	Teaspoons (tsp) sugar/100g	Sucrose (g/100g)	Fructose (g/100g)	Glucose (g/100g)	Average portion size	Grams (g) sugar per average portion	Tsp sugar per average portion
Potatoes, old, potato wedges, with skin, cooked in oil, homemade	1.7	½	0.4	0.6	0.7	average portion (150g)	2.6	¾
Potatoes, old, raw, flesh only	0.9	¼	Tr	0.4	0.5	200g each	1.8	½
Potatoes, old, roasted	1.2	¼	Tr	0.5	0.7	1 small potato (50g)	0.6	¼
						1 medium potato (85g)	1.0	¼
						1 large potato (130g)	1.6	½
						average portion (200g)	2.4	½
Potatoes, old, wedges, with skin, homemade, cooked in oil	1.7	½	0.4	0.6	0.7	average portion (150g)	2.6	¾
Sweet potato, baked	14.5	3¾	N	N	N	2 potatoes (130g)	18.9	4¾
Sweet potato, boiled in water, flesh only	11.6	3	N	N	N	2 potatoes (130g)	15.1	3¾
Sweet potato, raw, flesh only	5.7	1½	4.4	0.6	0.7	230g each	13.1	3¼
Sweet potato, steamed	8.4	2	N	N	N	2 potatoes (130g)	10.9	2¾

Poultry

Food name	Total sugars (g/100g)	Teaspoons (tsp) sugar/100g	Sucrose (g/100g)	Fructose (g/100g)	Glucose (g/100g)	Average portion size	Grams (g) sugar per average portion	Tsp sugar per average portion
Chicken breast in crumbs, chilled, fried	0.8	¼	N	N	N	1 Kiev (170g)	1.4	¼
Chicken breast/steak, coated, baked	1.1	¼	0.3	Tr	0.3	100g	1.1	¼
Chicken roll	0.0	0	0.0	0.0	0.0	1 slice (19g)	0.0	0
Chicken slices	0.2	0	0.2	0.0	0.0	1 thin slice (11g)	0.0	0
Chicken wings, marinated, meat and skin, barbecued, weighed with bone	2.3	½	1.6	0.4	0.3	5 wings (161g)	3.7	1
Chicken, breast, casseroled	0.0	0	0.0	0.0	0.0	small (180g) medium (260g) large (360g)	0.0 0.0' 0.0	0 0 0
Chicken, breast	0.0	0	0.0	0.0	0.0	large (150g) each	0.0	0
Chicken, breast, strips, stir-fried in oil	0.0	0	0.0	0.0	0.0	15g per strip	0.0	0
Chicken, drumsticks	0.0	0	0.0	0.0	0.0	with bone (90g) edible portion (47g)	0.0 0.0	0 0
Chicken, leg quarter	0.0	0	0.0	0.0	0.0	with bone (165g) edible portion (90g)	0.0 0.0	0 0
Chicken, portions, not coated, deep-fried	0.0	0	0.0	0.0	0.0	70g per piece	0.0	0
Chicken, thighs	0.0	0	0.0	0.0	0.0	with bone (75g) edible portion (45g)	0.0 0.0	0 0
Chicken, whole	0.0	0	0.0	0.0	0.0	700g (edible portion)	0.0	0
Chicken, wings	0.0	0	0.0	0.0	0.0	with bone (55g) edible portion (25g)	0.0 0.0	0 0
Chicken/turkey pieces, coated, baked	1.1	¼	0.4	Tr	0.2	70g per piece	0.8	¼
Duck, meat only, raw	0.0	0	0.0	0.0	0.0	1 whole 200g leg	0.0	0
Giblets, chicken or turkey	0.0	0	0.0	0.0	0.0	4oz (113g)	0.0	0
Goose, meat	0.0	0	0.0	0.0	0.0	700g raw weight	0.0	0
Grouse, meat	0.0	0	0.0	0.0	0.0	1 whole 400g bird	0.0	0
Liver, chicken, fried	0.0	0	0.0	0.0	0.0	100g	0.0	0
Partridge, roasted	0.0	0	0.0	0.0	0.0	small portion (120g)	0.0	0
Pheasant, roasted or casseroled	0.0	0	0.0	0.0	0.0	small portion (120g)	0.0	0

Food name	Total sugars (g/100g)	Teaspoons (tsp) sugar/100g	Sucrose (g/100g)	Fructose (g/100g)	Glucose (g/100g)	Average portion size	Grams (g) sugar per average portion	Tsp sugar per average portion
Pigeon, roasted	0.0	0	0.0	0.0	0.0	small portion (120g)	0.0	0
Poussin	0.0	0	0.0	0.0	0.0	1 whole 450g bird	0.0	0
Turkey slices	0.4	0	N	N	N	1 thin slice (11g)	0.0	0
Turkey, breast	0.0	0	0.0	0.0	0.0	½ 500g breast joint (250g)	0.0	0
Turkey, drumsticks	0.0	0	0.0	0.0	0.0	½ 1 whole 813g raw drumstick, 305g cooked	0.0 0.0	0 0
Turkey, meat	0.0	0	0.0	0.0	0.0	¼ 500g pack (125g)	0.0	0
Turkey, mince, stewed	0.0	0	0.0	0.0	0.0	¼ 500g pack (125g)	0.0	0
Turkey roll	0.0	0	0.0	0.0	0.0	1 slice (19g)	0.0	0
Turkey, self-basting, roasted	0.0	0	0.0	0.0	0.0	small portion (70g) medium portion (90g) large portion (140g)	0.0 0.0 0.0	0 0 0
Turkey, strips, stir-fried in oil	0.0	0	0.0	0.0	0.0	15g per strip	0.0	0
Turkey, thighs, diced, casseroled	0.0	0	0.0	0.0	0.0	small portion (70g) medium portion (90g) large portion (140g)	0.0 0.0 0.0	0 0 0

Puddings and ice cream

Food name	Total sugars (g/100g)	Teaspoons (tsp) sugar/100g	Sucrose (g/100g)	Fructose (g/100g)	Glucose (g/100g)	Average portion size	Grams (g) sugar per average portion	Tsp sugar per average portion
Arctic roll	25.3	6¼	16.9	1.1	2.6	1 slice, 1 fifth (50g)	12.7	3¼
Banana split, homemade	18.4	4½	8.7	2.3	4.3	180g	33.1	8¼
Blancmange, homemade	11.7	3	7.3	0.0	Tr	150g	17.6	4½
Bread pudding, homemade	33.3	8¼	12.2	8.5	8.9	190g	63.3	15¾
Cheese pudding, homemade	3.1	¾	N	N	N	170g	5.3	1¼
Chocolate nut sundae	29.9	7½	7.9	8.8	9.7	128g	38.3	9½
Coco fritters, fried in oil, homemade (West Indian dish)	0.9	¼	0.1	0.1	0.5	120g	1.1	¼
Coconut ice, homemade	67.1	31¾	66.0	0.2	Tr	60g	40.3	10
Cornetto type ice cream cone	27.9	7	19.1	1.5	2.0	81g each	22.6	5¾
Crème caramel, homemade	28.7	7¼	26.3	0.0	Tr	90g	25.8	6½
Creme caramel, retail	18.0	4½	10.3	1.3	2.3	128g	23.0	5¾
Crumble, apple, homemade	23.4	5¾	18.2	3.9	1.3	170g	39.8	10
Crumble, fruit, homemade	21.1	5¼	18.1	1.6	1.3	170g	35.9	9
Crumble, fruit, retail	21.8	5½	11.3	4.2	4.1	170g	37.1	9¼
Crumble, fruit, wholemeal, homemade	21.3	5¼	18.2	1.6	1.3	170g	36.2	9
Crumble, with pie filling, homemade	19.4	4¾	11.9	3.8	3.6	170g	33.0	8¼
Custard powder	Tr	Tr	Tr	0.0	Tr	1 whole 75g packet	Tr	0
Custard, egg	10.9	2¾	6.2	0.0	Tr	110g	12	3
Custard, made up with semi-skimmed milk	11.2	2¾	5.9	0.0	Tr	120g	13.4	3¼
Custard, made up with skimmed milk	11.3	2¾	5.9	0.0	Tr	120g	13.6	3½
Custard, made up with whole milk	11.1	2¾	5.9	0.0	Tr	120g	13.3	3¼
Custard, ready to eat, canned and tetra-pak	12.8	3¼	8.2	Tr	Tr	150g pot	19.2	4¾
Desserts, dairy, chocolate	24.0	6	17.3	0.2	0.4	80g each	19.2	4¾
Desserts, rice, with fruit, individual, chilled	13.6	3½	7.1	1.2	1.4	200g each	27.2	6¾
Dessert powder, instant	40.7	10¼	38.3	Tr	Tr	1 whole 59g packet	24.0	6

Food name	Total sugars (g/100g)	Teaspoons (tsp) sugar/100g	Sucrose (g/100g)	Fructose (g/100g)	Glucose (g/100g)	Average portion size	Grams (g) sugar per average portion	Tsp sugar per average portion
Dream Topping, made up with semi-skimmed milk	9.9	2½	4.4	Tr	Tr	3 dessertspoons (50g)	5.0	1¼
Dream Topping, made up with skimmed milk	9.6	2½	4.4	Tr	Tr	3 dessertspoons (50g)	4.8	1¼
Dream Topping, made up with whole milk	9.7	2½	4.4	Tr	Tr	3 dessertspoons (50g)	4.9	1¼
Dream Topping, powder	29.9	7½	21.5	Tr	Tr	1 whole 33g packet	9.9	2½
Fruit fool, homemade	16.1	4	13.4	0.9	0.8	120g	19.3	4¾
Gulab jamen/jambu, homemade	35.6	9	28.7	Tr	Tr	150g	53.4	13¼
Gulab jamen/jambu, retail	38.9	9¾	29.6	Tr	Tr	120g	46.7	12
Halva (Greek sweet)	53.1	13¼	N	N	N	150g	79.7	20
Halva, carrot, homemade	43.3	10¾	33.8	2.2	2.6	120g	52.0	13
Halva, semolina, homemade	37.6	9½	37.6	Tr	Tr	150g	56.4	14
Halwa (Asian sweet)	59.0	14¾	N	N	N	120g	70.8	17¾
Ice cream bars/choc ices, chocolate coated, luxury	32.9	8¼	23.9	1.5	1.4	57g each	18.8	4¾
Ice cream bars/choc ices, non-dairy, with chocolate flavoured coating	20.5	5	13.1	Tr	0.3	99g each	20.3	5
Ice cream desserts, frozen	19.7	5	13.8	Tr	0.5	1 thin slice (56g)	11.0	2¾
Ice cream sauce, topping, strawberry and chocolate flavours	62.3	15½	6.2	28.0	28.0	28g	17.4	4¼
Ice cream with cone, non-dairy, vanilla	22.6	5¾	11.1	0.8	4.8	91g each	20.6	5¼
Ice cream with wafers, non-dairy, vanilla	22.7	5¾	11.1	0.8	4.8	56g	12.7	3¼
Ice cream, dairy free/soya alternative	21.3	5¼	13.1	1.6	5.3	1 scoop (40g)	8.5	2¼
Ice cream, dairy, chocolate	24.2	6	17.3	Tr	2.6	1 scoop (40g)	9.7	2½
Ice cream, dairy, flavoured	23.7	6	12.3	1.5	5.2	1 scoop (40g)	9.5	2½
Ice cream, dairy, luxury, with chocolate/caramel	28.4	7	22.2	1.2	1.2	1 scoop (40g)	11.4	2¾
Ice cream, dairy, premium	16.7	4¼	12.0	Tr	Tr	1 scoop (40g)	6.7	1¾
Ice cream, dairy, vanilla, soft scoop	22.0	5½	11.9	0.9	2.7	1 scoop (40g)	8.8	2¼
Ice cream, non-dairy, chocolate	20.3	5	11.3	Tr	4.0	1 scoop (40g)	8.1	2

Food name	Total sugars (g/100g)	Teaspoons (tsp) sugar/100g	Sucrose (g/100g)	Fructose (g/100g)	Glucose (g/100g)	Average portion size	Grams (g) sugar per average portion	Tsp sugar per average portion
Ice cream, non-dairy, fruit flavoured	21.8	5½	10.4	0.9	5.2	1 scoop (40g)	8.7	2¼
Ice cream, non-dairy, vanilla, soft scoop	23.5	5¾	11.4	0.8	5.0	1 scoop (40g)	9.4	2¼
Ice cream, virtually fat free alternative	19.0	4¾	10.4	Tr	1.9	1 scoop (40g)	7.6	2
Ice Magic sauce, assorted chocolate flavours	29.4	7¼	29.4	Tr	Tr	28g	8.2	2
Instant dessert powder, made up with semi-skimmed milk (Angel Delight and own brand)	11.0	2¾	6.7	Tr	Tr	120g	13.2	3¼
Instant dessert powder, made up with skimmed milk	11.0	2¾	6.7	Tr	Tr	120g	13.2	3¼
Instant dessert powder, made up with whole milk	10.9	2¾	6.7	Tr	Tr	120g	13.1	3¼
Jelly, made with semi-skimmed milk	16.8	4¼	8.3	1.7	3.4	115g	19.3	4¾
Jelly, made with skimmed milk	16.8	4¼	8.3	1.7	3.4	115g	19.3	4¾
Jelly, made with water	15.1	3¾	8.6	1.7	3.5	115g	17.4	4¼
Jelly, made with whole milk	16.7	4¼	8.3	1.7	3.4	115g	19.2	4¾
Jelly, sugar free, made with water	0.0	0	0.0	0.0	0.0	115g	0.0	0
Knickerbocker glory, homemade	14.1	3½	8.0	1.2	2.5	180g	25.4	6¼
Kulfi, homemade	13.6	3½	0.3	4.4	3.6	80g	10.9	2¾
Lollies, containing ice-cream	20.9	5¼	12.6	0.4	2.9	77g each	16.1	4
Lollies, with real fruit juice	17.8	4½	15.9	0.9	1.0	57g each	10.1	2½
Meringue, homemade	96.0	24	96.0	0.0	Tr	8g each	7.7	2
Meringue, with cream, homemade	27.2	6¾	25.6	0.0	Tr	28g each	7.6	2
Mousse, chocolate	17.5	4¼	10.8	1.8	1.1	74g	8.2	2
Mousse, chocolate, low fat	15.8	4	3.8	6.3	Tr	74g	11.7	3
Mousse, fruit	18.0	4½	7.6	2.9	3.1	74g	13.3	3½
Pancakes, sweet, made with semi skimmed milk, homemade	17.0	4¼	13.8	Tr	Tr	small (60g) medium (110g) large (150g)	10.2 18.7 25.5	2½ 4¾ 6½
Pancakes, sweet, made with skimmed milk, homemade	17.0	4¼	13.8	Tr	Tr	small (60g) medium (110g) large (150g)	10.2 18.7 25.5	2½ 4¾ 6½

Food name	Total sugars (g/100g)	Teaspoons (tsp) sugar/100g	Sucrose (g/100g)	Fructose (g/100g)	Glucose (g/100g)	Average portion size	Grams (g) sugar per average portion	Tsp sugar per average portion
Pancakes, sweet, made with whole milk, homemade	16.9	4¼	13.8	Tr	Tr	small (60g) medium (110g) large (150g)	10.1 18.6 25.4	2½ 4¾ 6¼
Pavlova, toffee/chocolate, no fruit	45.3	11¼	40.1	0.8	2.1	100g	45.3	11¼
Pavlova, with fruit and cream	41.0	10¼	35.9	1.7	2.5	100g	41.0	10¼
Peach melba, homemade	14.9	3¾	6.8	1.8	3.3	150g	22.4	5½
Pie, apple, one crust, homemade	18.0	4½	12.7	3.8	1.4	110g	19.8	5
Pie, apple, pastry top and bottom, homemade	13.6	3½	9.4	2.8	1.1	110g	15.0	3¾
Pie, apple, pastry, double crust, deep filled, retail	18.0	4½	11.5	3.5	1.9	110g	19.8	5
Pie, apple, pastry, double crust, retail	7.0	1¾	4.6	1.3	1.1	110g	7.7	2
Pie, apple, wholemeal, one crust, homemade	18.0	4½	12.8	3.8	1.3	110g	19.8	5
Pie, apple, wholemeal, pastry top and bottom, homemade	13.7	3½	9.7	2.8	1.0	110g	15.1	3¾
Pie, banoffee	20.9	5¼	15.0	1.3	1.4	120g	25.1	6¼
Pie filling, fruit, assorted flavours	14.6	3¾	3.9	5.5	5.2	1 whole large can (395g)	57.7	14½
Pie, fruit, individual, retail	31.0	7¾	17.1	2.4	8.3	small (54g) large (100g)	16.7 31.0	4¼ 7¾
Pie, fruit, one crust, homemade	15.7	4	12.6	1.6	1.4	110g	17.3	4¼
Pie, fruit, pastry top and bottom, blackcurrant, homemade	12.5	3	9.1	1.6	1.6	110g	13.8	3½
Pie, fruit, pastry top and bottom, homemade	12.0	3	9.4	1.2	1.1	110g	13.2	3¼
Pie, fruit, wholemeal, one crust, homemade	15.8	4	12.8	1.6	1.3	110g	17.4	4¼
Pie, fruit, wholemeal, pastry top and bottom, blackcurrant, homemade	12.6	4¼	9.4	1.6	1.4	110g	13.9	3½
Pie, fruit, wholemeal, pastry top and bottom, homemade	12.1	3	9.7	1.2	1.0	110g	13.3	3¼
Pie, fruit, wholemeal, with pie filling, homemade	8.1	2	2.4	2.9	2.7	110g	8.9	2¼
Pie, fruit, with pie filling, homemade	8.1	2	2.0	2.9	2.9	110g	8.9	2¼

Food name	Total sugars (g/100g)	Teaspoons (tsp) sugar/100g	Sucrose (g/100g)	Fructose (g/100g)	Glucose (g/100g)	Average portion size	Grams (g) sugar per average portion	Tsp sugar per average portion
Pie, lemon meringue, retail	29.3	7¼	20.0	3.4	4.5	1 slice (150g)	44.0	11
Pinni, homemade	40.9	10¼	40.9	Tr	Tr	120g	49.1	12¼
Profiteroles with sauce, frozen	17.0	4¼	11.7	0.8	1.8	155g	26.4	6½
Pudding, bread and butter, homemade	12.4	3	4.7	1.5	1.6	170g	21.1	5¼
Pudding, Christmas, homemade	33.8	8½	N	N	N	100g	33.8	8½
Pudding, Christmas, retail	46.2	11½	3.5	20.8	20.3	100g	46.2	11½
Pudding, Eve's pudding, homemade	20.0	5	15.9	3.0	1.0	110g	22.0	5½
Pudding, Queen of Puddings, homemade	27.5	6¾	21.3	1.4	2.5	110g	30.3	7½
Pudding, rice, canned	8.7	2¼	4.9	Tr	Tr	small can (213g)	18.5	4¾
Pudding, rice, canned, low fat	8.7	2¼	4.9	Tr	Tr	small can (213g)	18.5	4¾
Pudding, rice, homemade, with semi-skimmed milk	10.3	2½	5.3	Tr	Tr	200g	20.6	5¼
Pudding, rice, homemade, with skimmed milk	10.4	2½	5.3	Tr	Tr	200g	20.8	5¼
Pudding, rice, homemade, with whole milk	10.2	2½	5.3	Tr	Tr	200g	20.4	5
Pudding, sponge, canned	25.8	6½	14.9	3.8	4.6	small individual pudding (100g)	25.8	6½
Pudding, sponge, homemade	18.5	4½	18.0	Tr	Tr	110g	20.4	5
Pudding, sponge, with dried fruit, homemade	25.2	6¼	16.5	4.1	4.1	110g	27.7	7
Pudding, sponge, with jam or treacle, homemade	25.8	6½	19.5	2.3	3.0	110g	28.4	7
Pudding, spotted dick, homemade	19.1	3¾	11.1	3.0	3.0	110g	21.0	5¼
Pudding, suet, homemade	14.5	3½	12.1	0.1	0.1	90g	13.1	3¼
Rum baba, homemade	19.7	5	19.7	Tr	Tr	198g	39.0	9¾
Seviyan, homemade	13.6	3½	8.3	0.5	0.5	120g	16.3	4
Sorbet, fruit	23.3	5¾	17.2	1.6	3.6	95g	22.1	5½
Tiramisu	21.1	5¼	13.5	1.4	2.3	90g	19.0	4¾
Torte, fruit	17.4	4¼	13.0	0.6	1.3	95g	16.5	4¼
Treacle tart, homemade	33.8	8½	13.7	9.6	9.8	95g	32.1	8
Trifle, chocolate, individual	2.3	½	0.0	0.0	0.0	105g	2.4	½

Food name	Total sugars (g/100g)	Teaspoons (tsp) sugar/100g	Sucrose (g/100g)	Fructose (g/100g)	Glucose (g/100g)	Average portion size	Grams (g) sugar per average portion	Tsp sugar per average portion
Trifle, fruit, retail	15.3	3¾	6.2	4.6	1.8	113g	17.3	4¼
Trifle, homemade	16.7	4½	8.9	2.0	2.7	170g	28.4	7
Trifle, with Dream Topping	17.1	4¼	9.2	2.0	2.7	170g	29.1	7¼
Wafers, plain ice cream wafers, not filled	3.5	¾	3.5	Tr	Tr	2g each 1 fan (5g)	0.1 0.2	0 0
Waffles, homemade	3.4	¾	0.2	Tr	Tr	65g	2.2	½

Rice, noodles and pasta

Food name	Total sugars (g/100g)	Teaspoons (tsp) sugar/100g	Sucrose (g/100g)	Fructose (g/100g)	Glucose (g/100g)	Average portion size	Grams (g) sugar per average portion	Tsp sugar per average portion
Cannelloni, spinach, homemade	2.0	¼	0.1	0.1	0.1	100g each	2	½
Cannelloni, vegetable, homemade	2.4	¼	0.2	0.2	0.2	100g each	2.4	½
Lasagne, homemade	2.8	¾	0.3	0.4	0.5	420g	11.8	3
Lasagne, retail, reheated	3.0	¾	0.4	0.7	0.6	400g	12	3
Lasagne, spinach, wholemeal, homemade	2.2	½	0.3	0.4	0.5	420g	9.2	2 ¼
Lasagne, vegetable, retail	4.4	1	0.2	0.7	0.7	420g	18.5	4¾
Lasagne, vegetable, wholemeal, homemade	3.0	¾	0.3	0.7	0.8	420g	12.6	3¼
Macaroni cheese, canned	1.9	½	0.9	0.1	0.1	large tin (430g) small tin (210g)	8.2 4.0	2 1
Macaroni cheese, homemade	2.8	¾	0.1	0.0	0.0	average portion (220g)	6.2	1½
Noodles, egg, dried, raw	1.7	½	0.6	0.2	0.2	¼ 350g packet (93g)	1.6	½
Noodles, egg, fine, dried, boiled in water	Tr	0	Tr	Tr	Tr	280g	Tr	0
Noodles, egg, fried with spring onions, homemade	0.2	0	0.0	0.1	0.1	280g	0.6	¼
Noodles, egg, medium, dried, boiled in water	Tr	0	Tr	Tr	Tr	280g	Tr	0
Noodles, egg, thick, dried, boiled in water	Tr	0	Tr	Tr	Tr	280g	Tr	0
Noodles, rice, fine, dried, boiled in water	Tr	0	Tr	Tr	Tr	280g	Tr	0
Pasta and sauce mixes, dried, raw	8.1	2	1.2	0.5	0.4	110g packet	8.9	2¼
Pasta shapes, coloured, flavoured, dried, raw	2.3	½	0.3	0.3	0.2	small portion (75g) large portion (115g)	1.7 2.6	½ ¾
Pasta with ham and mushroom sauce, homemade	1.0	¼	Tr	0.1	Tr	470g	4.7	1¼
Pasta with meat and tomato sauce, homemade	1.9	½	0.2	0.7	0.7	470g	8.9	2¼
Pasta, egg, fresh, filled with cheese and tomato, boiled in water	0.2	0	Tr	0.2	Tr	470g	0.9	¼

Food name	Total sugars (g/100g)	Teaspoons (tsp) sugar/100g	Sucrose (g/100g)	Fructose (g/100g)	Glucose (g/100g)	Average portion size	Grams (g) sugar per average portion	Tsp sugar per average portion
Pasta, egg, fresh, filled with cheese only, boiled in water	2.2	½	Tr	Tr	Tr	470g	10.3	2½
Pasta, egg, fresh, filled with green vegetables/herbs and cheese, boiled in water	0.1	0	Tr	0.1	Tr	470g	0.5	¼
Pasta, egg, fresh, filled with meat, boiled in water	1.0	¼	Tr	0.1	Tr	470g	4.7	1¼
Pasta, egg, fresh, filled with mushrooms, boiled in water	0.7	¼	Tr	Tr	Tr	470g	3.3	¾
Pasta, egg, fresh, raw	2.1	½	Tr	0.4	0.3	small portion (115g)	2.4	½
						large portion (150g)	3.2	¾
Pasta, egg, white, dried, raw	2.1	½	0.2	0.2	0.2	small portion (75g)	1.6	½
						large portion (115g)	2.4	½
Pasta, egg, white, tagliatelle, fresh, boiled in water	Tr	0	Tr	Tr	Tr	small portion (150g)	Tr	0
						medium portion (230g)	Tr	0
						large portion (350g)	Tr	0
Pasta, plain, fresh, boiled	0.6	¼	0.1	0.0	0.1	small portion (150g)	0.9	¼
						medium portion (230g)	1.4	¼
						large portion (350g)	2.1	½
Pasta, ravioli, meat filling, canned in tomato sauce	3.4	¾	1.1	0.9	1.0	small can (200g)	6.8	1¾
						large can (400g)	13.6	3½
Pasta, spaghetti, canned in bolognese sauce	2.5	¾	1.0	0.7	0.5	small can (200g)	5.0	1¼
						large can (400g)	10.0	2½
Pasta, spaghetti, canned, in tomato sauce	5.5	1¼	2.4	1.4	1.3	small can (200g)	11.0	2¾
						large can (400g)	22.0	5½
Pasta, white, twists, fusilli, dried, boiled in water	0.6	¼	Tr	Tr	Tr	small portion (150g)	0.9	¼
						medium portion (230g)	1.4	¼
						large portion (350g)	2.1	½

Food name	Total sugars (g/100g)	Teaspoons (tsp) sugar/100g	Sucrose (g/100g)	Fructose (g/100g)	Glucose (g/100g)	Average portion size	Grams (g) sugar per average portion	Tsp sugar per average portion
Pasta, white, dried, boiled in water	1.1	¼	0.2	0.1	0.1	small portion (150g)	1.7	½
						medium portion (230g)	2.5	¾
						large portion (350g)	3.9	1
Pasta, white, dried, raw	2.1	½	0.3	0.2	0.1	small portion (75g)	1.6	½
						large portion (115g)	2.4	½
Pasta, white, spaghetti, dried, boiled in water	1.0	¼	Tr	0.1	Tr	small portion (150g)	1.5	½
						medium portion (230g)	2.3	½
						large portion (350g)	3.5	1
Pasta, wholewheat, spaghetti, dried, boiled in water	Tr	0	Tr	Tr	Tr	small portion (150g)	Tr	0
						medium portion (230g)	Tr	0
						large portion (350g)	Tr	0
Pasta, wholewheat, spaghetti, dried, raw	3.9	1	0.5	0.4	0.4	small portion (75g)	2.9	¾
						large portion (115g)	4.5	1¼
Pilaf, rice with spinach, homemade	1.6	½	0.5	0.5	0.5	180g	2.9	¾
Pilaf, rice with tomato, homemade	0.9	¼	0.2	0.4	0.4	180g	1.6	½
Pilau, egg and potato, brown rice, homemade	1.6	½	0.6	0.4	0.6	180g	2.9	¾
Pilau, egg and potato, homemade	1.4	¼	0.5	0.4	0.5	180g	2.5	¾
Pilau, mushroom, homemade	0.8	¼	0.2	0.2	0.3	180g	1.4	¼
Pilau, prawn, homemade	0.8	¼	0.2	0.2	0.3	180g	1.4	¼
Pilau, vegetable, homemade	0.3	0	Tr	0.3	Tr	180g	0.5	¼
Pot savouries (noodles, rice and chilli)	8.2	2	3.9	1.9	1.3	180g each	14.8	3¾
Pot savouries, made up	2.3	½	1.1	0.5	0.4	300g each	6.9	1¾
Red rice, boiled in water	0.2	0	0.2	Tr	Tr	1 heaped tablespoon (40g)	0.1	0

Food name	Total sugars (g/100g)	Teaspoons (tsp) sugar/100g	Sucrose (g/100g)	Fructose (g/100g)	Glucose (g/100g)	Average portion size	Grams (g) sugar per average portion	Tsp sugar per average portion
Rice and black-eye beans	0.9	¼	0.5	0.1	0.1	220g	2.0	½
Rice and black-eye beans, brown rice	1.0	¼	0.8	0.1	0.3	220g	2.2	½
Rice and pigeon peas	0.7	¼	0.4	0.1	0.1	220g	1.5	½
Rice and pigeon peas, brown rice	0.8	¼	0.6	0.1	0.3	220g	1.8	½
Rice and red kidney beans	0.5	¼	0.4	0.0	0.0	220g	1.1	¼
Rice and red kidney beans, brown rice	0.6	¼	0.6	0.0	0.2	220g	1.3	¼
Rice and split peas	0.8	¼	0.4	0.1	0.1	220g	1.8	½
Rice and split peas, brown rice	0.9	¼	0.7	0.1	0.3	220g	2.0	½
Rice, brown, basmati, boiled in water	0.3	0	0.3	Tr	Tr	1 heaped tablespoon (40g)	0.1	0
Rice, brown, basmati, raw	0.8	¼	0.8	Tr	Tr	75g	0.6	¼
Rice, brown, easy cook, boiled in water	0.3	0	0.3	Tr	Tr	1 heaped tablespoon (40g)	0.1	0
Rice, brown, easy cook, raw	0.7	¼	0.6	Tr	0.1	75g	0.5	¼
Rice, brown, wholegrain, boiled in water	0.1	0	0.1	Tr	Tr	1 heaped tablespoon (40g)	0.0	0
Rice, brown, wholegrain, raw	0.7	¼	0.7	Tr	Tr	75g	0.5	¼
Rice, egg fried, ready cooked, re-heated, retail, not takeaway	Tr	0	Tr	Tr	Tr	270g	Tr	0
Rice, pilau, plain, homemade	0.8	¼	0.3	0.2	0.3	180g	1.4	¼
Rice, ready-cooked, "plain", re-heated	Tr	0	Tr	Tr	Tr	1 heaped tablespoon (40g)	Tr	0
Rice, red, raw	0.9	¼	0.8	Tr	Tr	75g	0.7	¼
Rice, savoury, including chicken, beef, mushroom and vegetable varieties, dried, cooked	3.2	¾	1.4	0.5	0.5	300g each	9.6	2½
Rice, savoury, including chicken, beef, mushroom and vegetable varieties, dried, uncooked	6.7	1¾	3.3	1.1	0.9	180g each	12.1	3
Rice, Thai fragrant, boiled in water	Tr	0	Tr	Tr	Tr	1 heaped tablespoon (40g)	Tr	0
Rice, Thai fragrant, raw	0.1	0	Tr	Tr	Tr	1 heaped tablespoon (40g)	0.0	0
Rice, white, basmati, boiled in water	Tr	0	Tr	Tr	Tr	1 heaped tablespoon (40g)	Tr	0

Food name	Total sugars (g/100g)	Teaspoons (tsp) sugar/100g	Sucrose (g/100g)	Fructose (g/100g)	Glucose (g/100g)	Average portion size	Grams (g) sugar per average portion	Tsp sugar per average portion
Rice, white, basmati, easy cook, boiled in water	Tr	0	Tr	Tr	Tr	1 heaped tablespoon (40g)	Tr	0
Rice, white, basmati, easy cook, raw	0.6	¼	0.5	Tr	Tr	75g	0.5	¼
Rice, white, basmati, raw	0.1	0	0.1	Tr	Tr	75g	0.1	0
Rice, white, Italian "Arborio" risotto, boiled in water	Tr	0	Tr	Tr	Tr	1 heaped tablespoon (40g)	Tr	0
Rice, white, Italian Arborio risotto, raw	0.2	0	0.2	Tr	Tr	75g	0.2	0
Rice, white, long grain, boiled in water	Tr	0	Tr	Tr	Tr	1 heaped tablespoon (40g)	Tr	0
Rice, white, long grain, easy cook, boiled in water	Tr	0	Tr	Tr	Tr	1 heaped tablespoon (40g)	Tr	0
Rice, white, long grain, easy cook, raw	Tr	0	Tr	Tr	Tr	75g	Tr	0
Rice, white, long grain, raw	0.2	0	0.2	Tr	Tr	75g	0.2	0
Rice, white, pudding, raw	0.2	0	0.2	Tr	Tr	75g	0.2	0
Rice, wild, boiled in water	0.4	0	0.3	Tr	Tr	1 heaped tablespoon (40g)	0.3	0
Rice, wild, raw	0.1	0	0.1	Tr	Tr	75g	0.1	0
Risotto, plain, homemade	1.0	¼	0.4	0.3	0.3	400g	4.0	1
Risotto, vegetable, brown rice	1.8	½	0.7	0.5	0.5	400g	7.2	1¾
Risotto, white rice, vegetable, homemade	1.7	½	0.6	0.5	0.5	400g	6.8	1¾
Spaghetti bolognese, homemade	1.8	½	0.2	0.6	0.6	470g	8.5	2¼
Spaghetti bolognese, retail, meat and sauce only, reheated	3.0	¾	0.6	1.3	1.1	400g	12.0	3
Spaghetti bolognese, retail, reheated, with spaghetti	1.9	½	0.3	0.6	0.5	400g	7.6	2
Tagliatelle, with vegetables, retail	2.2	½	0.9	0.5	0.5	400g	8.8	2¼
Turkey and pasta bake, homemade	2.0	½	0.1	0.4	0.3	430g	8.6	2¼

Salads and light meals

Food name	Total sugars (g/100g)	Teaspoons (tsp) sugar/100g	Sucrose (g/100g)	Fructose (g/100g)	Glucose (g/100g)	Average portion size	Grams (g) sugar per average portion	Tsp sugar per average portion
Bhaji, aubergine and potato, homemade	3.2	¾	0.7	1.1	1.4	30g each	1.0	¼
Bhaji, aubergine, pea, potato and cauliflower, homemade	4.3	1	2.6	0.8	0.9	30g each	1.3	¼
Bhaji, cabbage and pea, homemade	7.1	1¾	2.8	2.0	2.3	30g each	2.1	½
Bhaji, cabbage and pea, with rapeseed oil, homemade	7.1	1¾	2.8	2.0	2.3	30g each	2.1	½
Bhaji, cabbage and potato, with butter, homemade	4.9	1¼	0.6	2.0	2.3	30g each	1.5	½
Bhaji, cabbage and potato, with rapeseed oil, homemade	4.7	1¼	0.7	1.9	2.2	30g each	1.4	¼
Bhaji, cabbage, homemade	5.9	1½	0.9	2.3	2.6	30g each	1.8	½
Bhaji, carrot, potato and pea, with butter, homemade	6.8	1¾	4.2	1.2	1.3	30g each	2.0	½
Bhaji, carrot, potato and pea, with vegetable oil, homemade	6.7	1¾	4.2	1.2	1.3	30g each	2.0	½
Bhaji, cauliflower and potato, homemade	2.8	¾	0.4	1.3	1.2	30g each	0.8	¼
Bhaji, cauliflower and vegetable, homemade	4.0	1	0.5	1.6	1.6	30g each	1.2	¼
Bhaji, cauliflower, homemade	3.8	1	0.6	1.6	1.5	30g each	1.1	¼
Bhaji, karela, homemade	Tr	0	Tr	Tr	Tr	30g each	Tr	0
Bhaji, mushroom, homemade	3.2	¾	1.0	1.0	1.1	30g each	1.0	¼
Bhaji, mustard leaves and spinach, homemade	1.6	½	0.3	0.5	0.6	30g each	0.5	¼
Bhaji, mustard leaves, homemade	1.3	¼	0.1	0.5	0.6	30g each	0.4	0
Bhaji, okra, Bangladeshi, homemade	5.6	1½	1.9	1.7	1.9	30g each	1.7	½
Bhaji, okra, Islami, homemade	7.0	1¾	2.2	2.4	2.3	30g each	2.1	½

Food name	Total sugars (g/100g)	Teaspoons (tsp) sugar/100g	Sucrose (g/100g)	Fructose (g/100g)	Glucose (g/100g)	Average portion size	Grams (g) sugar per average portion	Tsp sugar per average portion
Bhaji, pea, homemade	3.2	¾	1.8	0.5	0.7	30g each	1.0	¼
Bhaji, potato and green pepper, homemade	2.6	¾	0.3	1.2	1.1	30g each	0.8	¼
Bhaji, potato and onion, homemade	3.4	¾	1.2	0.9	1.2	30g each	1.0	¼
Bhaji, potato, onion and mushroom, homemade	3.5	1	1.2	1.0	1.3	30g each	1.1	¼
Bhaji, potato, spinach and cauliflower, homemade	1.6	½	0.5	0.5	0.6	30g each	0.5	¼
Bhaji, potato, homemade	1.5	½	0.6	0.4	0.5	30g each	0.5	¼
Bhaji, spinach and potato, homemade	1.6	½	0.6	0.5	0.5	30g each	0.5	¼
Bhaji, spinach, homemade	2.1	½	0.7	0.7	0.7	30g each	0.6	¼
Bhaji, turnip and onion, homemade	5.9	1½	1.4	2.0	2.6	30g each	1.8	½
Bhaji, turnip, homemade	5.4	1¼	0.8	2.0	2.7	30g each	1.7	½
Bhaji, vegetable, with butter, homemade	4.7	1¼	1.4	1.5	1.8	30g each	1.4	¼
Bhaji, vegetable, with oil, homemade	4.6	1¼	1.4	1.5	1.8	30g each	1.4	¼
Chicken/turkey pasties/slices, puff pastry	1.2	¼	0.2	0.1	0.2	125g each	1.5	¼
Corn fritters, fried in oil, homemade (West Indian dish)	4.9	1¼	3.3	0.2	0.3	130g	6.4	1½
Cornish pasty, homemade	2.3	½	0.6	0.6	0.9	medium (145g) large (227g)	3.3 5.2	¾ 1¼
Cornish pasty, retail	2.1	½	0.4	0.4	0.5	medium (155g) large (260g)	3.3 5.5	¾ 1¼
Coronation chicken, homemade	3.4	¾	1.3	0.7	1.1	115g	3.9	1
Coronation chicken, reduced fat, homemade	2.9	¾	1.1	0.9	0.8	115g	3.3	¾
Dosa, filling, vegetable, homemade	4.1	1	0.9	1.4	1.6	30g	1.3	¼
Falafel, fried in oil, homemade	2.7	¾	1.3	0.6	0.8	16g each	0.4	0

Food name	Total sugars (g/100g)	Teaspoons (tsp) sugar/100g	Sucrose (g/100g)	Fructose (g/100g)	Glucose (g/100g)	Average portion size	Grams (g) sugar per average portion	Tsp sugar per average portion
Flan, cheese and mushroom, homemade	2.2	½	0.1	0.1	0.2	1 slice (120g)	2.6	¾
Flan, cheese and mushroom, wholemeal, homemade	2.3	½	0.3	0.1	0.1	1 slice (120g)	2.8	¾
Flan, cheese, onion and potato, homemade	1.0	¼	0.2	0.2	0.3	1 slice (120g)	1.2	¼
Flan, cheese, onion and potato, wholemeal, homemade	1.0	¼	0.4	0.2	0.2	1 slice (120g)	1.2	¼
Flan, lentil and tomato, homemade	2.5	¾	0.8	0.8	0.9	1 slice (120g)	3.0	¾
Flan, lentil and tomato, wholemeal, homemade	2.6	¾	0.8	0.8	0.9	1 slice (120g)	3.1	¾
Flan, spinach, homemade	1.8	½	0.2	0.2	0.3	1 slice (120g)	2.2	½
Flan, spinach, wholemeal, homemade	1.9	½	0.4	0.2	0.3	1 slice (120g)	2.3	½
Flan, vegetable, homemade	2.7	¾	0.8	0.4	0.6	1 slice (120g)	3.2	¾
Flan, vegetable, wholemeal, homemade	2.7	¾	1.0	0.4	0.5	1 slice (120g)	3.2	¾
Pakora/bhajia, aubergine, fried, homemade	2.1	½	0.8	0.6	0.8	50g each	1.1	¼
Pakora/bhajia, cauliflower, fried, homemade	2.8	¾	1.0	0.9	0.8	50g each	1.4	¼
Pakora/bhajia, onion, fried, homemade	3.4	¾	1.8	0.7	0.8	50g each	1.7	½
Pakora/bhajia, potato and cauliflower, fried, homemade	2.0	½	1.0	0.4	0.5	50g each	1.0	¼
Pakora/bhajia, potato, carrot and pea, fried, homemade	1.9	½	1.6	0.1	0.1	50g each	1.0	¼
Pakora/bhajia, potato, fried, homemade	1.4	¼	0.8	0.3	0.3	50g each	0.7	¼
Pakora/bhajia, spinach, fried, homemade	1.9	½	1.5	0.2	0.2	50g each	1.0	¼

Food name	Total sugars (g/100g)	Teaspoons (tsp) sugar/100g	Sucrose (g/100g)	Fructose (g/100g)	Glucose (g/100g)	Average portion size	Grams (g) sugar per average portion	Tsp sugar per average portion
Pakora/bhajia, vegetable, retail	2.4	½	1.1	0.6	0.7	50g each	1.2	¼
Pakoras, homemade	2.1	½	1.0	0.5	0.6	50g each	1.1	¼
Pancakes, stuffed with vegetables, homemade	4.4	1	0.4	1.0	1.1	145g	6.4	1½
Pancakes, stuffed with vegetables, wholemeal, homemade	4.5	1¼	0.5	1.0	1.1	145g	6.5	1¾
Pasty, vegetable, homemade	1.8	½	0.7	0.3	0.5	125g each	2.3	½
Pasty, vegetable, wholemeal, homemade	1.9	½	1.0	0.3	0.3	125g each	2.4	½
Pie, pork and egg	1.3	¼				140g	1.8	1
Pizza, cheese and tomato, French bread, retail	2.4	½	0.2	0.7	0.5	1 individual pizza (160g)	3.8	1
Pizza, cheese and tomato, retail	3.9	1	Tr	0.9	0.8	**Deep pan:**		
						1 slice of 12" (87.5g)	3.4	¾
						1 slice of 10" (68g)	2.7	¾
						individual 7" (230g)	9.0	2¼
						Thin crust:		
						1 slice of 12" (70g)	2.7	¾
						1 slice of 10" (43g)	1.7	½
						individual 7" (116g)	4.5	1¼
Pizza, chicken topped, retail	2.1	½	Tr	0.7	0.5	**Deep pan:**		
						1 slice of 12" (100g)	2.1	½
						1 slice of 10" (83g)	1.7	½
						individual 7" (290g)	6.1	1½
						Thin crust:		
						1 slice of 12" (82.5g)	1.7	½
						1 slice of 10" (52g)	1.1	¼
						individual 7" (150g)	3.2	¾
Pizza, ham and pineapple, retail	3.1	¾	Tr	0.8	0.7	**Deep pan:**		
						1 slice of 12" (100g)	3.1	¾
						1 slice of 10" (83g)	2.6	¾
						individual 7" (290g)	9.0	2¼
						Thin crust:		
						1 slice of 12" (82.5g)	2.6	¾
						1 slice of 10" (52g)	1.6	½
						individual 7" (150g)	4.7	1¼

Food name	Total sugars (g/100g)	Teaspoons (tsp) sugar/100g	Sucrose (g/100g)	Fructose (g/100g)	Glucose (g/100g)	Average portion size	Grams (g) sugar per average portion	Tsp sugar per average portion
Pizza, tomato, homemade	3.0	¾	0.8	1.1	1.0	Deep pan:		
						1 slice of 12" (100g)	3.0	¾
						1 slice of 10" (83g)	2.5	¾
						individual 7" (300g)	9.0	2¼
						Thin crust:		
						1 slice of 12" (82.5g)	2.5	¾
						1 slice of 10" (57g)	1.7	½
						individual 7" (150g)	4.5	1¼
Pizza, tomato, wholemeal, homemade	3.2	¾	1.0	1.1	1.0	Deep pan:		
						1 slice of 12" (100g)	3.2	¾
						1 slice of 10" (83g)	2.7	¾
						individual 7" (300g)	9.6	1½
						Thin crust:		
						1 slice of 12" (82.5g)	2.6	¾
						1 slice of 10" (57g)	1.8	½
						individual 7" (150g)	4.8	1¼
Pork pie, individual	1.5	½	0.1	Tr	0.2	buffet pie (75g)	1.1	¼
						individual (140g)	2.1	½
Pork pie, sliced	0.0	0				60g	0.0	0
Quiche, cheese and egg, homemade	1.6	½	Tr	Tr	0.1	¼ (95g)	1.5	½
						mini (40g)	0.6	¼
Quiche, cheese and egg, wholemeal, homemade	1.6	½	0.2	Tr	Tr	¼ (95g)	1.5	½
						mini (40g)	0.6	¼
Quiche, Lorraine, homemade	2.2	½	Tr	Tr	0.1	¼ (95g)	2.1	½
						mini (40g)	0.9	¼
Quiche, Lorraine, shortcrust pastry, retail	3.2	¾	0.3	0.3	0.4	¼ (95g)	3.0	¾
						mini (40g)	1.3	¼
Quiche, Lorraine, wholemeal pastry, homemade	2.2	½	0.2	Tr	Tr	¼ (95g)	2.1	½
						mini (40g)	0.9	¼
Quiche, mushroom, homemade	1.3	¼	Tr	0.1	0.1	¼ (95g)	1.2	¼
						mini (40g)	0.5	¼
Quiche, mushroom, wholemeal, homemade	1.3	¼	0.2	0.1	Tr	¼ (95g)	1.2	¼
						mini (40g)	0.5	¼
Quiche, vegetable, retail	3.5	1	0.2	0.4	0.6	¼ (95g)	3.3	¾
						mini (40g)	1.4	¼
Rissoles, brown rice, fried	1.5	½	N	N	N	40g each	0.6	¼
Rissoles, chick pea, fried	0.4	0	0.4	0.0	0.0	40g each	0.2	0
Rissoles, lentil, fried	2.0	½	N	N	N	40g each	0.8	¼

Food name	Total sugars (g/100g)	Teaspoons (tsp) sugar/100g	Sucrose (g/100g)	Fructose (g/100g)	Glucose (g/100g)	Average portion size	Grams (g) sugar per average portion	Tsp sugar per average portion
Rissoles, vegetable, fried	1.6	½	0.8	0.4	0.4	40g each	0.6	¼
Salad, bean with French dressing, retail	2.6	¾	1.8	0.4	0.4	200g	5.2	1¼
Salad, beetroot and onion in French dressing	8.2	2	N	N	N	200g	16.4	4
Salad, carrot and nut with French dressing, retail	13.2	3¼	3.5	4.7	5.0	200g	26.4	6½
Salad, carrot and nut with mayonnaise, retail	9.4	2¼	2.3	3.0	3.1	200g	18.8	4¾
Salad, Florida, retail	9.6	2½	2.3	2.8	3.2	200g	19.2	4¾
Salad, Greek	1.8	½	0.0	0.9	0.7	200g	3.6	1
Salad, green (lettuce, cucumber, pepper and celery)	1.6	½	0.0	0.9	0.7	200g	3.2	¾
Salad, potato, with reduced calorie dressing, retail	4.0	1	3.8	0.1	0.2	200g	8.0	2
Salad, pasta, vegetables and mayonnaise	1.9	½	1.0	0.5	0.4	200g	3.8	1
Salad, potato, with French dressing	2.1	½	N	N	N	200g	4.2	1
Salad, potato, with mayonnaise	1.5	½	0.7	0.4	0.4	200g	3.0	¾
Salad, potato, with mayonnaise, retail	1.9	0.5	1.3	0.2	0.4	200g	3.8	1
Salad, rice, brown (rice, vegetables, nut and raisin)	5.0	1¼	1.1	1.9	2.0	200g	10.0	2½
Salad, rice, homemade (rice, vegetables, nut and raisin)	4.9	1¼	1.0	1.9	2.0	200g	9.8	2½
Salad, tomato and onion	4.1	1	N	N	N	200g	8.2	2
Salad, vegetable, canned	6.7	1¾	5.0	0.8	0.8	200g	13.4	3¼
Salad, Waldorf	7.9	2	2.2	4.3	1.4	200g	15.8	4
Salad, Waldorf, retail	8.4	2	1.2	3.8	3.3	200g	16.8	4¼

Food name	Total sugars (g/100g)	Teaspoons (tsp) sugar/100g	Sucrose (g/100g)	Fructose (g/100g)	Glucose (g/100g)	Average portion size	Grams (g) sugar per average portio	Tsp sugar per avera
Salad, wholemeal pasta, with vegetables and mayonnaise	2.6	¾	0.9	0.6	0.7	200g	5.2	1¼
Samosas, lamb, baked, homemade	1.6	½	0.6	0.3	0.4	75g each	3.2	¾
Samosas, lamb, deep fried, homemade	1.2	¼	0.4	0.2	0.3	75g each	0.9	¼
Samosas, vegetable, retail	2.7	¾	1.1	0.2	0.3	75g each	2.0	½
Sausage roll, flaky pastry, ready-to-eat, retail	1.3	¼	0.2	Tr	0.2	mini cocktail (14g) small (32g) medium (60g) large/jumbo (145g)	0.2 0.4 0.8 1.9	0 0 ¼ ½
Sausage rolls, short pastry, homemade	2.1	½	0.0	Tr	0.8	mini cocktail (14g) medium (60g)	0.3 1.3	 ¼
Scotch eggs, retail	Tr	0	0.0	0.0	Tr	average (120g) mini, picnic (60g)	Tr Tr	0 0
Tabouleh	0.7	¼	0.0	0.3	0.3	250g	1.8	½
Welsh rarebit, homemade	2.4	½	Tr	0.1	Tr	1 slice (67g)	1.6	½
Welsh rarebit, wholemeal, homemade	2.1	½	Tr	0.2	0.1	1 slice (67g)	1.4	¼

Sauces and condiments

Food name	Total sugars (g/100g)	Teaspoons (tsp) sugar/100g	Sucrose (g/100g)	Fructose (g/100g)	Glucose (g/100g)	Average portion size	Grams (g) sugar per average portion	Tsp sugar per average portion
Apple sauce, homemade	20.2	5	13.7	4.8	1.6	20g	4.0	1
Barbecue sauce	29.9	7.5	N	N	N	1 tablespoon (25g)	7.5	2
Barbecue sauce, homemade	21.5	5½	17.1	2.0	1.8	1 tablespoon (25g)	5.4	1¼
Black bean sauce	11.1	2¾	6.4	2.6	2.1	1 tablespoon (20g)	2.2	½
Bread sauce, made with semi-skimmed milk, homemade	5.4	1¼	0.5	0.5	0.6	45g	2.4	½
Bread sauce, made with skimmed milk, homemade	5.1	1¼	0.5	0.4	0.6	45g	2.3	½
Bread sauce, made with whole milk, homemade	5.0	1¼	0.5	0.4	0.5	45g	2.3	½
Brown fruity sauce	19.6	5	4.0	8.3	7.3	1 sachet (12g)	2.4	½
						1 portion pack (20g)	3.9	1
Brown sauce	24.2	6	8.7	8.0	7.5	1 sachet (12g)	2.9	¾
						1 portion pack (20g)	4.8	1¼
Brown sauce, reduced salt/ sugar	14.1	3.5	3.0	5.9	5.2	1 sachet (12g)	1.7	½
						1 portion pack (20g)	2.8	¾
Cheese sauce, made with semi-skimmed milk, homemade	4.2	1	0.0	Tr	Tr	small portion (30g)	1.3	¼
						medium portion (62g)	2.6	¾
						large portion (90g)	3.8	1
Cheese sauce, made with skimmed milk, homemade	4.3	1	0.0	Tr	Tr	small portion (30g)	1.3	¼
						medium portion (62g)	2.7	¾
						large portion (90g)	3.9	1
Cheese sauce, made with whole milk, homemade	4.1	1	0.0	Tr	Tr	small portion (30g)	1.2	¼
						medium portion (62g)	2.5	¾
						large portion (90g)	3.7	1

Food name	Total sugars (g/100g)	Teaspoons (tsp) sugar/100g	Sucrose (g/100g)	Fructose (g/100g)	Glucose (g/100g)	Average portion size	Grams (g) sugar per average portion	Tsp sugar per average portion
Cheese sauce, packet mix, made up with semi-skimmed milk, homemade	5.3	1¼	0.0	Tr	Tr	small portion (30g)	1.6	½
						medium portion (62g)	3.3	¾
						large portion (90g)	4.8	1¼
Cheese sauce, packet mix, made up with skimmed milk, homemade	5.3	1¼	0.0	Tr	Tr	small portion (30g)	1.6	½
						medium portion (62g)	3.3	¾
						large portion (90g)	4.8	1¼
Cheese sauce, packet mix, made up with whole milk, homemade	5.1	1¼	0.0	Tr	Tr	small portion (30g)	1.5	½
						medium portion (62g)	3.2	¾
						large portion (90g)	4.6	1¼
Chilli sauce	6.9	1¾	Tr	3.8	3.1	1 teaspoon (6g)	0.4	0
Chutney, apple, homemade	48.4	12	38.4	5.7	4.3	1 teaspoon (10g)	4.8	1¼
						1 tablespoon (33g)	16.0	4
Chutney, mango, oily	49.1	12¼	N	N	N	1 teaspoon (10g)	4.9	1¼
						1 tablespoon (33g)	16.2	4
Chutney, mango, sweet	45.7	11½	5.6	19.5	20.6	1 teaspoon (10g)	4.6	1¼
						1 tablespoon (33g)	15.1	3¾
Chutney, mixed fruit	37.4	9¼	3.4	17.2	16.8	1 teaspoon (10g)	3.7	1
						1 tablespoon (33g)	12.3	3
Chutney, tomato	28.1	7	0.3	14.2	13.6	1 teaspoon (10g)	2.8	¾
						1 tablespoon (33g)	9.3	2¼
Chutney, tomato, homemade	40.2	10	32.3	4.0	3.8	1 teaspoon (10g)	4.0	1
						1 tablespoon (33g)	13.3	3¼
Coleslaw, not low calorie, retail	6.0	1½	3.5	1.2	1.4	1 tablespoon (45g)	2.7	¾
Coleslaw, with reduced calorie dressing, retail	6.5	1¾	3.7	1.3	1.6	1 tablespoon (45g)	2.9	¾
Coleslaw, with vinaigrette, retail	12.2	3	8.6	1.6	1.8	1 tablespoon (45g)	5.5	1½
Cranberry sauce	39.3	9¾	3.5	17.9	17.9	30g	11.8	3

Food name	Total sugars (g/100g)	Teaspoons (tsp) sugar/100g	Sucrose (g/100g)	Fructose (g/100g)	Glucose (g/100g)	Average portion size	Grams (g) sugar per average portion	Tsp sugar per average portion
Dressing, blue cheese	7.7	2	0.2	3.5	4.0	1 tablespoon (25g)	1.9	½
Dressing, 'fat free', assorted flavours	10.3	2½	5.1	1.9	3.3	1 tablespoon (25g)	2.6	¾
Dressing, French	6.7	1.8	N	N	N	1 tablespoon (15g)	1.0	¼
Dressing, French, fat free	8.6	2¼	N	N	N	1 tablespoon (15g)	1.3	¼
Dressing, French, homemade	0.2	0	0.0	0.1	0.1	1 tablespoon (15g)	0.0	0
Dressing, low fat, assorted flavours	6.0	1½	N	N	N	1 tablespoon (25g)	1.5	½
Dressing, oil and lemon, homemade	3.4	¾	3.1	0.2	0.1	1 tablespoon (15g)	0.5	¼
Dressing, thousand island	13.4	3¼	N	N	N	1 tablespoon (30g)	4.0	1
Dressing, thousand island, reduced calorie	14.7	3¾	4.6	5.1	5.0	1 tablespoon (30g)	4.4	1
Dressing, yogurt, homemade	7.0	1¾	Tr	0.1	Tr	1 tablespoon (25g)	1.8	½
Gherkins, pickled, drained	2.4	½	1.1	0.8	0.5	1 small (8g)	0.2	
						1 large (25g)	0.6	¼
Gravy instant granules	5.3	1½	N	N	N	1 tsp (3g)	0.2	0
Gravy instant granules, made up with water	0.4	0	N	N	N	small average portion (25g)	0.1	0
						medium average portion (50g)	0.2	0
						large average portion (120g)	0.5	¼
Hollandaise sauce, homemade	0.5	¼	Tr	Tr	Tr	1 tablespoon (30g)	0.2	0
Horseradish sauce	15.0	3¾	7.4	3.6	4.0	1 sachet (12g)	1.8	½
						1 portion pack (20g)	3.0	¾
Hot pepper sauce	0.9	¼	Tr	0.5	0.4	1 tsp (5g)	0.0	0
Mayonnaise, homemade	0.1	0	Tr	Tr	Tr	1 heaped tablespoon (33g)	0.0	0
						1 level tablespoon (15g)	0.0	0
						1 portion pack (12g)	0.0	0

Food name	Total sugars (g/100g)	Teaspoons (tsp) sugar/100g	Sucrose (g/100g)	Fructose (g/100g)	Glucose (g/100g)	Average portion size	Grams (g) sugar per average portion	Tsp sugar per average portion
Mayonnaise, reduced fat	4.6	1¼	2.5	1.0	1.1	1 heaped tablespoon (33g)	1.5	½
Mayonnaise, standard, retail	2.4	½	1.7	0.4	0.3	1 heaped tablespoon (33g)	0.8	¼
Mint sauce	21.5	5½	11.8	4.8	4.9	average portion (10g) 1 teaspoon (7g)	2.2 1.5	½ ½
Mustard, smooth	7.8	2	1.5	2.9	3.4	average portion (2g) 1 sachet (5g)	0.2 0.4	0 0
Mustard, wholegrain	3.9	1	Tr	1.9	2.0	average portion (14g) 1 sachet (5g)	0.5 0.2	¼ 0
Onion sauce, made with semi-skimmed milk, homemade	4.8	1¼	0.5	0.4	0.6	62g	3.0	¾
Onion sauce, made with skimmed milk, homemade	4.8	1¼	0.5	0.4	0.6	62g	3.0	¾
Onion sauce, made with whole milk, homemade	4.8	1¼	0.4	0.3	0.4	62g	3.0	¾
Pesto, green	2.3	½	Tr	0.4	1.1	26g	0.6	¼
Pesto, red	5.2	1¼	N	N	N	26g	1.4	¼
Piccalilli	14.8	3¾	1.5	6.8	6.5	1 tablespoon (40g)	5.9	1½
Pickle, sweet	24.6	6¼	8.2	8.4	8.0	average portion (40g) 1 heaped teaspoon (15g) 1 tablespoon (40g) 1 portion pack (20g)	9.8 3.7 9.8 4.9	2½ 1 2½ 1¼
Raita, homemade	5.8	1½	Tr	0.2	0.2	1 tablespoon (45g)	2.6	¾
Raita, yogurt and gram flour, homemade	5.3	1¼	0.9	0.7	0.9	1 tablespoon (45g)	2.4	½
Relish, corn/cucumber/onion	28.9	7.3	10.5	9.4	9.0	1 heaped teaspoon (15g)	4.3	1
Relish, tomato based	25.1	6¼	11.8	6.8	6.5	in burger (15g) 1 heaped teaspoon (15g)	3.8 3.8	1 1
Salad cream	16.7	4¼	12.9	1.9	1.9	average with salad (20g) 1 sachet (12g)	3.3 2.0	¾ ½

Food name	Total sugars (g/100g)	Teaspoons (tsp) sugar/100g	Sucrose (g/100g)	Fructose (g/100g)	Glucose (g/100g)	Average portion size	Grams (g) sugar per average portion	Tsp sugar per average portion
Salad cream, reduced fat	9.2	2¼	4.4	2.3	2.5	average with salad (20g)	1.8	½
						1 sachet (12g)	1.1	¼
Sauce, cheese, packet mix, dry	5.6	1½	0.3	Tr	Tr	1 whole packet (40g)	2.2	½
Sauce, Chinese cook in, sweet & sour	19.4	4¾	9.7	4.8	4.8	½ 450g bottle (225g)	43.7	11
Sauce, Chinese stir fry	16.7	4¼	9.3	3.6	3.7	½ small 120g packet (60g)	10.0	2½
Sauce, curry, onion, with butter, homemade	4.4	1	1.4	1.2	1.6	150g	6.6	1¾
Sauce, curry, onion, with vegetable oil, homemade	4.2	1	1.4	1.2	1.6	150g	6.3	1½
Sauce, curry, sweet, UK type, homemade	5.7	1½	0.9	2.5	2.2	150g	8.6	2¼
Sauce, curry, tomato and onion, homemade (Gujerati dish)	4.6	1¼	0.7	1.9	2.0	150g	6.9	1¾
Sauce, dry, casserole mix (including liver and bacon, sausage, beef Bourguignon mixes)	12.2	3	4.8	2.3	3.8	¼ 40g packet (10g)	1.2	¼
Sauce, dry, casserole mix, made up	1.2	¼	0.5	0.2	0.4	small portion (30g)	0.4	0
						medium portion (62g)	0.7	¼
						large portion (90g)	1.1	¼
Sauce, dry mix	12.8	3¼	7.1	2.4	1.8	1 whole packet (40g)	5.1	1¼
Sauce, duck a l'orange	1.8	½	0.5	0.6	0.6	average portion (62g)	1.1	¼
Sauce, Indian cook in, korma/ tikka masala (ambient)	7.4	1¾	3.2	2.0	1.6	¼ 450g bottle (112.5g)	8.3	2
Sauce, pasta, carbonara type (chilled and ambient)	0.8	¼	Tr	Tr	Tr	½ 350g bottle (175g)	1.4	¼
Sauce, pasta, four cheese (chilled and ambient)	1.9	½	N	Tr	Tr	½ 350g bottle (175g)	3.3	¾
Sauce, pasta, tomato based, for bolognese (ambient)	6.1	1½	1.3	2.6	2.2	½ 350g bottle (175g)	10.7	2¾
Sauce, pasta, tomato based, napoletana (including tomato and basil sauce, ambient)	6.3	1½	0.7	2.7	2.9	½ 350g bottle (175g)	11.0	2¾

Food name	Total sugars (g/100g)	Teaspoons (tsp) sugar/100g	Sucrose (g/100g)	Fructose (g/100g)	Glucose (g/100g)	Average portion size	Grams (g) sugar per average portion	Tsp sugar per average portion
Sauce, pasta, tomato based, reduced fat (ambient)	5.6	1½	1.1	2.4	2.1	½ 350g bottle (175g)	9.8	2½
Sauce, pasta, tomato based, with added vegetables (including chargrilled vegetable, sweet pepper, arrabbiata and mushroom pasta sauce, ambient)	5.1	1¼	1.2	2.1	1.8	½ 350g bottle (175g)	8.9	1¼
Sauce, pasta, white, with ham and mushrooms, homemade	1.0	¼	0.1	0.1	0.1	medium portion (150g)	1.5	½
Sauce, sweet and sour, take-away (purchased from Chinese restaurants)	27.5	7	8.3	9.7	9.5	150g	41.2	10¼
Sauce, tomato and mushroom, homemade	4.7	1¼	0.7	1.9	2.0	90g	4.2	1
Sauce, tomato based, homemade	5.1	1¼	1.2	1.9	1.9	90g	4.6	1¼
Sauce, traditional cook in, tomato based (including chasseur and red wine sauce, chilled and ambient)	4.9	1¼	1.6	1.7	1.5	¼ 500g bottle (125g)	6.1	1½
Sauce, traditional cook in, white sauce based (including white wine sauces, cheese sauces and creamy sauces, chilled and ambient)	2.8	¾	1.2	0.5	0.5	¼ 500g bottle (125g)	3.5	1
Sauce, white, packet mix, dry	6.2	1½	2.5	Tr	Tr	1 whole packet (40g)	2.5	¾
Sauces, Indian cook in, other (including balti, rogan josh, jalfrezi, ambient)	6.1	1½	1.9	2.3	1.9	¼ 450g bottle (112.5g)	6.9	1¾
Soy sauce, light and dark varieties	16.4	4	9.6	2.0	4.8	1 teaspoon (5g)	0.8	¼
Tartare sauce	16.2	4	6.5	6.3	3.4	average serving (30g)	4.9	1¼
Tomato ketchup	27.5	7	15.2	6.4	5.9	1 sachet (12g)	1.9	½
						1 sachet (12g)	3.3	¾
						1 portion pack (20g)	5.5	1¼
Tomato sauce, homemade	4.0	1				90g	3.6	1
Vinegar	0.6	¼	0.0	0.3	0.3	1 teaspoon (5g)	0.0	0
						1 tablespoon (15g)	0.1	0

Food name	Total sugars (g/100g)	Teaspoons (tsp) sugar/100g	Sucrose (g/100g)	Fructose (g/100g)	Glucose (g/100g)	Average portion size	Grams (g) sugar per average portion	Tsp sugar per average portion
White sauce, packet mix, made up with semi-skimmed milk	5.2	1¼	0.2	Tr	Tr	small portion (30g)	1.6	½
						medium portion (62g)	3.2	¾
						large portion (90g)	4.7	1¼
White sauce, packet mix, made up with skimmed milk	5.2	1¼	0.2	Tr	Tr	small portion (30g)	1.6	½
						medium portion (62g)	3.2	¾
						large portion (90g)	4.7	1¼
White sauce, packet mix, made up with whole milk	5.0	1¼	0.2	Tr	Tr	small portion (30g)	1.5	½
						medium portion (62g)	3.1	¾
						large portion (90g)	4.5	1¼
White sauce, savoury, made with semi-skimmed milk, homemade	5.1	1¼	0.0	Tr	Tr	small (30g)	1.5	½
						medium (62g)	3.2	¾
						large (90g)	4.6	1¼
White sauce, savoury, made with skimmed milk, homemade	5.2	1¼	0.0	Tr	Tr	small (30g)	1.6	½
						medium (62g)	3.2	¾
						large (90g)	4.7	1¼
White sauce, savoury, made with whole milk, homemade	4.9	1¼	0.0	Tr	Tr	small (30g)	1.5	½
						medium (62g)	3.0	¾
						large (90g)	4.4	1¼
White sauce, sweet, made with semi-skimmed milk, homemade	13.2	3¼	8.6	Tr	Tr	small portion (30g)	4.0	1
						medium portion (62g)	8.2	2
						large portion (90g)	11.9	3
White sauce, sweet, made with skimmed milk, homemade	13.3	3¼	8.6	Tr	Tr	small portion (30g)	4.0	1
						medium portion (62g)	8.2	2
						large portion (90g)	12.0	3
White sauce, sweet, made with whole milk, homemade	13.1	3¼	8.6	Tr	Tr	small portion (30g)	3.9	1
						medium portion (62g)	8.1	2
						large portion (90g)	11.8	3
Worcestershire sauce	21.5	5½	N	N	N	1 teaspoon (5g)	1.1	¼

Snacks, dips
and crisps

Food name	Total sugars (g/100g)	Teaspoons (tsp) sugar/100g	Sucrose (g/100g)	Fructose (g/100g)	Glucose (g/100g)	Average portion size	Grams (g) sugar per average portion	Tsp sugar per average portion
Bombay mix	2.3	½	2.2	0.1	0.1	large bag (100g)	2.3	½
Cassava chips	5.5	1¼	4.0	0.7	0.7	35g	1.9	½
Chevra and chana chur	3.4	¾	N	N	N	30g	1.0	¼
Corn snacks (e.g. Wotsits, Monster Munch)	5.5	1¼	0.6	Tr	Tr	27g	1.5	½
Corn and starch snacks (Skips etc.)	4.2	1	3.5	0.2	0.5	18g	0.8	¼
Dips, sour-cream based, assorted flavours	2.0	½	0.4	0.7	0.9	1 heaped tablespoon (33g)	0.7	¼
Dips, sour-cream based, reduced fat	3.4	¾	Tr	N	N	1 heaped tablespoon (33g)	1.1	¼
Green beans, dried	22.6	5¾	Tr	14.4	8.2	30g	6.8	1¾
Guacamole, homemade	1.3	¼	0.1	0.6	0.6	1 tablespoon (15g)	0.2	0
Houmous	0.6	¼	0.5	0.1	Tr	1 tablespoon (15g)	0.1	0
Maize and rice flour snacks (Frazzles and Bacon Streaks)	1.6	½	0.7	Tr	0.9	27g	0.4	0
Mixed cereal and potato flour snacks (such as cheese balls)	1.4	¼	1.0	0.2	0.2	25g	0.4	0
Popcorn, candied	15.0	3¾	15.0	Tr	Tr	individual bag (80g)	12.0	3
Popcorn, salted, retail	0.6	¼	0.6	Tr	Tr	individual bag (80g)	0.5	¼
Pork scratchings	0.2	0	Tr	Tr	0.2	22g	0.0	0
Potato and corn sticks (e.g. chipsticks, crunchy sticks)	1.5	½	1.0	0.3	0.2	19g	0.3	0
Potato and tapioca snacks (assorted including Waffles, Bitza Pizza, Wickettes)	2.8	¾	2.0	0.4	0.4	25g	0.7	¼
Potato crisps, crinkle cut	0.9	¼	0.6	Tr	0.3	40g	0.4	0
Potato crisps, fried in vegetable oil	0.9	¼	0.9	Tr	Tr	30g	0.3	0
Potato crisps, jacket	0.7	¼	0.6	Tr	0.1	30g	0.2	0
Potato crisps, low fat	1.5	½	0.8	Tr	0.2	30g	0.5	¼
Potato crisps, square	1.9	½	0.7	0.3	0.2	29g	0.6	¼
Potato crisps, thick, crinkle-cut	0.5	¼	0.4	Tr	0.1	40g	0.2	0
Potato crisps, thick-cut	1.5	½	0.9	0.2	0.4	50g	0.8	¼

Food name	Total sugars (g/100g)	Teaspoons (tsp) sugar/100g	Sucrose (g/100g)	Fructose (g/100g)	Glucose (g/100g)	Average portion size	Grams (g) sugar per average portion	Tsp sugar per average portion
Potato rings (e.g. Hula Hoops)	0.3	0	0.3	Tr	Tr	30g	0.1	0
Potato snacks, pringle-type, fried in vegetable oil	1.5	½	1.1	0.2	0.3	tube (200g)	3.0	¾
Puffed potato products	2.2	½	0.7	0.1	0.3	25g	0.6	¼
Rice flour cakes, glutinous, Chinese	32.0	8	N	N	N	25g	8.0	2
Salami snack (Peperami and own brand equivalents)	1.9	½	0.0	0.0	1.9	25g each	0.5	¼
Sev/ganthia, homemade	1.9	½	1.9	Tr	Tr	35g	0.7	¼
Taramasalata	1.2	¼	N	N	N	1 tablespoon (45g)	0.5	¼
Tortilla chips fried in vegetable oil	2.5	¾	1.1	0.2	0.2	½ 200g bag (100g)	2.5	¾
Trail mix	37.1	9¼	3.4	16.1	17.3	75g	27.8	7
Twiglets	0.6	¼	0.6	Tr	Tr	50g	0.3	0
Tzatziki	3.0	¾	0.0	0.3	0.4	1 tablespoon (15g)	0.5	¼
Wheat crunchies	2.1	½	1.4	0.1	0.6	35g	0.7	¼

Soups and sandwiches

Food name	Total sugars (g/100g)	Teaspoons (tsp) sugar/100g	Sucrose (g/100g)	Fructose (g/100g)	Glucose (g/100g)	Average portion size	Grams (g) sugar per average por	Tsp sugar per ave
Bouillabaisse, homemade	1.7	½	0.4	0.5	0.6	1 bowl (340g)	5.8	1½
Consomme	0.1	0	Tr	0.1	Tr	small portion (150g)	0.2	0
						medium portion (220g)	0.2	0
						large portion (300g)	0.3	0
Coronation chicken, homemade	3.4	¾	1.3	0.7	1.1	115g	3.9	1
Coronation chicken, reduced fat, homemade	2.9	¾	1.1	0.9	0.8	115g	3.3	¾
Sandwich spread	20.1	5	N	N	N	30g	6.0	1½
Sandwich, white bread, bacon, lettuce and tomato	2.4	½	0.1	0.4	0.2	195g	4.7	1¼
Sandwich, white bread, cheddar cheese and pickle	4.6	1¼	0.9	1.1	0.9	185g	8.5	2¼
Sandwich, white bread, chicken salad	2.1	½	0.0	0.4	0.2	205g	4.3	1
Sandwich, white bread, egg mayonnaise	2.2	½	0.1	0.1	0.0	145g	3.2	¾
Sandwich, white bread, ham salad	2.5	¾	0.2	0.4	0.2	185g	4.6	1¼
Sandwich, white bread, tuna mayonnaise	2.1	½	0.1	0.1	0.0	165g	3.5	1
Scotch broth, homemade	1.6	½	0.6	0.5	0.6	small portion (150g)	2.4	½
						medium portion (220g)	3.5	1
						large portion (300g)	4.8	1¼
Soup, broccoli and stilton, carton, chilled	1.5	½	0.2	0.3	0.2	large carton (600g)	9.0	2¼
Soup, carrot and coriander, carton, chilled	3.0	¾	1.6	0.6	0.6	large carton (600g)	18.0	4½
Soup, carrot and orange, homemade	3.5	1	1.4	0.9	1.1	small portion (150g)	5.3	1¼
						medium portion (220g)	7.7	2
						large portion (300g)	10.5	2¾
Soup, chicken noodle, dried	4.4	1¼	3.5	0.5	0.4	76g	3.3	¾
Soup, chicken noodle, dried, as served	0.3	0	0.2	Tr	Tr	215g	0.6	¼
Soup, chicken, cream of, canned	1.1	¼	0.6	0.1	Tr	large can (405g)	4.5	1¼

Food name	Total sugars (g/100g)	Teaspoons (tsp) sugar/100g	Sucrose (g/100g)	Fructose (g/100g)	Glucose (g/100g)	Average portion size	Grams (g) sugar per average portion	Tsp sugar per average portion
Soup, chicken, cream of, canned, condensed	1.4	¼	0.4	0.2	Tr	1 can (295g)	4.1	1
Soup, cream of tomato, canned	5.5	1½	2.2	1.5	1.3	large can (405g)	22.3	5½
Soup, French onion, homemade	3.7	1	1.5	1.0	1.3	small portion (150g) medium portion (220g) large portion (300g)	5.6 8.1 11.1	1½ 2 2¾
Soup, gazpacho, homemade	2.5	¾	0.2	1.2	1.1	small portion (150g) medium portion (220g) large portion (300g)	3.8 5.5 7.5	1 1½ 2
Soup, goulash, homemade	1.9	½	0.4	0.7	0.8	small portion (150g) medium portion (220g) large portion (300g)	2.9 4.2 5.7	¾ 1 1½
Soup, instant, dried, as purchased	17.4	4¼	6.7	1.7	2.1	76g	13.2	3¼
Soup, instant, dried, as served	1.7	½	0.6	0.2	0.2	215g	3.7	1
Soup, lentil, canned	1.2	¼	Tr	0.7	0.5	large can (405g)	4.9	1¼
Soup, lentil, homemade	1.7	½	0.8	0.5	0.5	small portion (150g) medium portion (220g) large portion (300g)	2.6 3.7 5.1	¾ 1 1¼
Soup, low calorie, canned	2.4	½	Tr	1.2	1.2	large can (405g)	9.7	2½
Soup, minestrone, canned	1.8	½	N	N	N	large can (405g)	7.3	1¾
Soup, minestrone, dried	19.7	5	12.9	3.8	3.0	76g	15	3¾
Soup, minestrone, dried, as served	1.4	¼	0.9	0.3	0.2	215g	3	¾
Soup, minestrone, homemade	1.4	¼	0.4	0.5	0.5	small portion (150g) medium portion (220g) large portion (300g)	2.1 3.1 4.2	½ ¾ 1
Soup, mulligatawny, homemade	2.9	¾	0.6	1.1	1.1	small portion (150g) medium portion (220g) large portion (300g)	4.4 6.4 8.7	1 1½ 2¼
Soup, mushroom, carton, chilled	1.4	¼	0.3	0.2	0.1	large carton (600g)	8.4	2
Soup, mushroom, cream of, canned	0.8	¼	0.3	0.1	Tr	large can (405g)	3.2	¾
Soup, oxtail, canned	0.9	¼	0.5	0.2	0.2	large can (405g)	3.6	1
Soup, oxtail, dried	9.2	2¼	5.5	0.9	1.0	76g	7	1¾

Food name	Total sugars (g/100g)	Teaspoons (tsp) sugar/100g	Sucrose (g/100g)	Fructose (g/100g)	Glucose (g/100g)	Average portion size	Grams (g) sugar per average portion	Tsp sugar per average portion
Soup, oxtail, dried, as served	0.7	¼	0.4	0.1	0.1	215g	1.5	½
Soup, pea and ham, homemade	1.5	½	0.7	0.3	0.4	small portion (150g) medium portion (220g) large portion (300g)	2.3 3.3 4.5	½ ¾ 1¼
Soup, potato and leek, homemade	1.5	½	0.2	0.2	0.2	small portion (150g) medium portion (220g) large portion (300g)	2.3 3.3 4.5	½ ¾ 1¼
Soup powder, instant, reduced calorie, assorted flavours	5.0	1¼	3.3	0.9	0.8	76g	3.8	1
Soup powder, instant, reduced calorie, assorted flavours, as served	0.8	¼	0.5	0.1	0.1	215g	1.7	½
Soup, tomato, carton, chilled	3.3	¾	1.1	1.1	1.0	large carton (600g)	19.8	5
Soup, tomato, cream of, canned, condensed	11.2	2¾	6.2	1.8	2.4	1 can (295g)	33.0	8¼
Soup, tomato, dried	37.0	9¼	26.9	5.5	4.6	76g	28.1	7
Soup, tomato, dried, as served	3.4	¾	2.5	0.5	0.4	215g	7.3	1¾
Soup, vegetable, canned	2.6	¾	1.1	0.8	0.7	large can (405g)	10.5	2¾
Soup, vegetable, dried	11.6	3	6.3	2.8	2.5	76g	8.8	2¼
Soup, vegetable, dried, as served	0.9	¼	0.5	0.2	0.2	215g	1.9	½
Soup, vegetable, homemade	1.8	½	0.8	0.5	0.5	small portion (150g) medium portion (220g) large portion (300g)	2.7 4.0 5.4	¾ 1 1¼
Soup, Wholesoup, canned	1.2	¼	Tr	0.7	0.5	large can (405g)	4.9	1¼

Sweets and confectionery

Food name	Total sugars (g/100g)	Teaspoons (tsp) sugar/100g	Sucrose (g/100g)	Fructose (g/100g)	Glucose (g/100g)	Average portion size	Grams (g) sugar per average portion	Tsp sugar per average portion
Bounty bar and own brand equivalents	50.4	12½	41.7	0.1	3.2	twin (57g) mini (29g)	28.7 14.6	7¼ 3¾
Burfi (Indian fudge-type sweet)	1.2	¼	N	N	N	1 inch square (11g)	0.1	0
Caramel bars and sweets, chocolate covered	56.0	14	39.6	Tr	4.7	bar (50g) treat size (17g)	28.0 9.5	7 2½
Chocolate covered bar with caramel and cereal	46.4	11½	32.9	Tr	2.1	standard bar (51g) treat size (19g)	23.7 8.8	6 2¼
Chocolate covered caramel and biscuit fingers	45.4	11¼	31.6	Tr	4.5	6g each	2.7	¾
Chocolate covered wafer biscuit	45.1	11¼	38.2	Tr	Tr	19g	8.6	2¼
Chocolate nut spread	59.7	15	56.7	Tr	Tr	1 heaped teaspoon (16g) 1 level teaspoon (8g)	9.6 4.8	2½ 1¼
Chocolate spread	59.4	14¾	49.5	Tr	Tr	1 heaped teaspoon (16g) 1 level teaspoon (8g)	9.5 4.8	2½ 1¼
Chocolate, cooking	55.9	14	55.9	Tr	Tr	200g bar	111.8	28
Chocolate, dark, with crème or mint fondant centres	62.9	15¾	56.5	2.4	4.0	8g each (i.e. After Eights)	5.0	1¼
Chocolate, fancy and filled	60.0	15	45.7	3.1	5.4	8g each (from a box of chocolates)	4.8	1¼
Chocolate, milk	56.0	14	46.8	Tr	Tr	standard bar (54g) square (7g) miniature (5g)	30.2 3.9 2.8	7½ 1 ¾
Chocolate, plain	62.6	15¾	62.4	Tr	Tr	small bar (50g)	31.3	7¾
Chocolate, white	58.3	14½	47.6	Tr	Tr	chunky bar (37g) small bar (13g)	21.6 7.6	5½ 2
Creme egg	58.0	14½	45.7	1.8	3.6	standard (39g) mini (12g)	22.6 7.0	5¾ 1¾
Fruit gums/jellies (i.e. wine gums)	58.7	14¾	46.4	Tr	6.3	each (3g)	1.8	½
Fruit pastilles	59.3	14¾	45.4	2.1	6.5	each (2g)	1.2	¼
Fudge, homemade	80.8	20¼	75.7	0.0	0.0	1 inch square (11g)	8.9	2¼

Food name	Total sugars (g/100g)	Teaspoons (tsp) sugar/100g	Sucrose (g/100g)	Fructose (g/100g)	Glucose (g/100g)	Average portion size	Grams (g) sugar per average portion	Tsp sugar per average portion
Gajjeralla	39.3	9¾	32.8	1.1	1.1	50g	19.7	5
Liquorice allsorts	55.5	14	36.9	Tr	2.3	each (5g)	2.8	¾
Liquorice shapes	41.5	10½	27.7	5.4	5.0	each (3g)	1.2	¼
Maltesers and similar products	63.3	15¾	38.7	0.3	7.8	each (2g)	1.2	¼
Mars bar and own brand equivalents	64.5	16¼	41.5	0.7	12.1	kingsize (100g) standard (65g) funsize (19g)	64.5 41.9 12.2	16¼ 10½ 3
Marshmallows	48.7	12¼	48.6	0.0	0.0	each (5g)	2.4	½
Marzipan, homemade	67.6	17	62.2	1.1	2.7	30g	20.3	5
Marzipan, white and yellow, retail	67.6	17	62.2	1.1	2.7	250g pack	155.5	39
Milky Way and own brand equivalents	69.7	17	47.1	0.3	6.5	standard (26g) funsize (17g)	18.1 11.8	4½ 3
Nougat, homemade	79.6	20	72.6	3.8	3.2	10g per sweet	8.0	2
Peanut brittle, homemade	71.8	18	64.2	3.8	3.8	bar (58g)	41.6	10½
Peppermint creams, homemade	95.9	24	95.9	Tr	Tr	6g each	5.8	1½
Peppermints	102.7	25¾	101.7	0.0	1.0	5g each	5.1	1¼
Smartie-type sweets	70.8	17¾	65.6	Tr	0.3	tube (37g) mini box (15g)	26.2 10.6	6½ 2¾
Sweets, boiled	86.7	21¾	67.5	1.4	8.5	7g each	6.1	1½
Sweets, chew sweets (Starburst, Chewits and Blackjacks)	54.5	13¾	40.5	Tr	6.3	3g each	1.6	½
Sweets, foam sweets	72.3	18	60.0	2.0	4.7	3g each	2.2	½
Sweets, sherbert (Refreshers, Parma Violets, Fizzers and Love Hearts)	93.9	23½	93.7	Tr	0.2	1g each	0.9	¼
Toffees, mixed	39.1	9¾	29.9	Tr	5.9	8g each	3.1	¾
Topic/Snickers and own brand equivalents	46.1	11½	31.0	0.1	4.8	king size (100g) standard (61g) fun size (19g)	46.1 28.1 8.8	11½ 7 2¼
Truffles, mocha, homemade	62.9	15¾	60.1	Tr	Tr	10g each	6.3	1½
Truffles, rum, homemade	53.4	13¼	53.1	Tr	Tr	10g each	5.3	1¼
Turkish delight, with nuts, homemade	81.8	20½	81.8	Tr	Tr	1 square (15g)	12.3	3
Turkish delight, without nuts	68.6	17¼	N	N	N	chocolate covered bar (51g)	35.0	8¾

Takeaway food

Food name	Total sugars (g/100g)	Teaspoons (tsp) sugar/100g	Sucrose (g/100g)	Fructose (g/100g)	Glucose (g/100g)	Average portion size	Grams (g) sugar per average portion	Tsp sugar per average portion
Bhaji, cabbage and potato, with vegetable oil	4.9	1¼	0.6	2.0	2.3	35g	1.7	½
Bhaji, cabbage and spinach	3.8	1	0.9	1.4	1.6	35g	1.3	¼
Bhaji, cauliflower, potato and pea	2.5	¾	0.3	1.0	1.1	35g	0.9	¼
Bhaji, green bean	4.1	1	0.4	2.0	1.6	35g	1.4	¼
Bhaji, vegetable, Punjabi	5.5	1½	1.9	1.7	1.9	35g	1.9	½
Biryani, chicken, takeaway	0.9	¼	0.2	0.5	0.2	400g	3.6	1
Burger, Big Mac, takeaway	3.9	1	N	N	N	204g	8.0	2
Burger, cheeseburger, takeaway	5.7	1½	N	N	N	118g	6.7	1¾
Burger, hamburger, takeaway	6.6	1¾	N	N	N	106g	7.0	1¾
Burger, Quarter Pounder with cheese, takeaway	5.5	1¼	N	N	N	195g	10.7	2¾
Burger, Whopper, takeaway	4.2	1	N	N	N	258g	10.8	2¾
Chicken pieces, coated, takeaway	Tr	0	Tr	Tr	Tr	6 nuggets (105g)	Tr	0
Chicken portions, battered, deep fried, takeaway	0.0	0	0.0	0.0	0.0	1 breast portion (70g) 1 drumstick (131g) 1 wing (73g)	0.0 0.0 0.0	0 0 0
Chicken satay, takeaway	1.6	½	Tr	1.1	0.5	400g	6.4	1½
Chow mein, chicken, takeaway	0.3	0	Tr	0.3	Tr	350g	1.1	¼
Cod, in batter, fried, takeaway	1.0	¼	0.3	0.2	0.1	small portion (170g)	1.7	½
Curry, chicken, average, takeaway	1.2	¼	0.0	0.5	0.4	350g	4.2	1
Curry, chicken, Thai green, takeaway and restaurant	0.5	¼	Tr	0.5	Tr	350g	1.8	½
Curry, Prawn bhuna, takeaway	1.2	¼	Tr	0.7	0.5	350g	4.2	1
Curry, Prawn madras, takeaway	1.2	¼	0.1	0.4	0.5	350g	4.2	1

Food name	Total sugars (g/100g)	Teaspoons (tsp) sugar/100g	Sucrose (g/100g)	Fructose (g/100g)	Glucose (g/100g)	Average portion size	Grams (g) sugar per average portion	Tsp sugar per average portion
Curry, prawn, takeaway	1.4	¼	0.1	0.6	0.5	350g	4.9	1¼
Curry, Thai, stir-fry vegetable, takeaway and restaurant	1.6	½	Tr	0.8	0.8	3–4 tablespoons (200g)	3.2	¾
Curry, vegetable, takeaway	3.1	¾	0.9	1.1	1.1	3–4 tablespoons (200g)	6.2	1½
Doner kebab in pitta bread with salad	1.1	¼	Tr	0.3	0.3	small (220g) large (320g)	2.4 3.5	½ 1
Doner kebabs, meat only	0.0	0	0.0	0.0	0.0	small (85g) large 130g)	0.0 0.0	0 0
Fajita, chicken, meat only, takeaway and restaurant	Tr	0	Tr	Tr	Tr	360g	Tr	0
Meat samosas, takeaway	1.9	½	Tr	0.5	Tr	75g each	1.4	¼
Milkshake, thick, takeaway	11.1	2¾	1.4	4.2	0.3	small drink 250ml (268g) medium drink 400ml (428g) large drink 500ml (535g)	29.7 47.5 59.4	7½ 12 14¾
Nachos, cheese, takeaway	Tr	0	Tr	Tr	Tr	65g	Tr	0
Pakora, vegetable, takeaway and restaurant	1.5	½	0.7	0.6	0.2	35g	0.5	¼
Pakora/bhajia, onion, retail, takeaway	7.8	2	4.5	1.7	1.7	35g	2.7	¾
Pancakes (served with crispy duck), pancakes only, takeaway	5.2	1¼	0.4	Tr	0.1	125g	6.5	1½
Pizza, cheese and tomato, takeaway	2.3	½	Tr	0.6	0.4	Deep pan: 1 slice of 12" (87.5g) 1 slice of 10" (68g) individual 7" (230g) Thin crust: 1 slice of 12" (70g) 1 slice of 10" (43g) individual 7" (116g)	2.0 1.6 5.3 1.6 1.0 2.7	½ ½ 1¼ ½ ¼ ¾

Food name	Total sugars (g/100g)	Teaspoons (tsp) sugar/100g	Sucrose (g/100g)	Fructose (g/100g)	Glucose (g/100g)	Average portion size	Grams (g) sugar per average portion	Tsp sugar per average portion
Pizza, fish topped, takeaway	2.0	½	Tr	0.4	0.3	**Deep pan:**		
						1 slice of 12" (100g)	0.0	0
						1 slice of 10" (83g)	1.7	½
						individual 7" (290g)	5.8	2¼
						Thin crust:		
						1 slice of 12" (82.5g)	1.7	½
						1 slice of 10" (52g)	1.0	¼
						individual 7" (150g)	3.0	¾
Pizza, meat topped, retail and takeaway	1.8	½	Tr	0.5	0.4	**Deep pan:**		
						1 slice of 12" (100g)	0.0	0
						1 slice of 10" (83g)	1.5	½
						individual 7" (290g)	5.2	1¼
						Thin crust:		
						1 slice of 12" (82.5g)	1.5	½
						1 slice of 10" (52g)	0.9	¼
						individual 7" (150g)	2.7	¾
Pizza, vegetarian, retail and takeaway	2.4	½	Tr	0.7	0.6	**Deep pan:**		
						1 slice of 12" (100g)	0.0	0
						1 slice of 10" (83g)	2.0	½
						individual 7" (300g)	7.2	1½
						Thin crust:		
						1 slice of 12" (82.5g)	2.0	½
						1 slice of 10" (57g)	1.4	¼
						individual 7" (150g)	3.6	1
Pork, spare ribs, Chinese barbecue, takeaway	0.0	0	0.0	0.0	0.0	340g	0.0	0
Potato chips, fine cut, from fast food outlets	0.3	0	0.3	Tr	Tr	small portion (77g)	0.2	0
						medium portion (110g)	0.3	0
						large portion (155g)	0.5	¼
Potato chips, fried, from takeaway fish and chip shops	0.6	¼	0.3	0.1	0.1	small portion (210g)	1.3	¼
Prawn crackers, takeaway	2.2	½	1.9	Tr	Tr	70g	1.5	½
Rice, egg fried, takeaway	Tr	0	Tr	Tr	Tr	270g	Tr	0
Saveloy, unbattered, takeaway	1.3	¼	0.3	0.1	0.4	65g	0.8	¼
Sesame prawn toast, takeaway	0.8	¼	Tr	Tr	Tr	70g each	0.6	¼
Spring rolls, meat, takeaway	1.8	½	0.5	0.6	0.4	60g each	1.1	¼

Food name	Total sugars (g/100g)	Teaspoons (tsp) sugar/100g	Sucrose (g/100g)	Fructose (g/100g)	Glucose (g/100g)	Average portion size	Grams (g) sugar per average portion	Tsp sugar per average portion
Stir-fry beef with green peppers and blackbean sauce, takeaway	1.0	¼	Tr	0.7	0.3	360g	3.6	1
Sweet and sour chicken, takeaway	10.7	2¾	4.1	3.2	3.4	300g	32.1	8
Sweet and sour pork, battered, takeaway	11.5	3	4.2	3.6	3.7	150g	17.3	4¼
Szechuan prawns with vegetables, takeaway	0.8	¼	Tr	0.4	0.4	340g	2.7	¾
Vegetable pancake roll, Chinese style, takeaway	3.0	¾	1.4	0.8	0.8	small (90g) large (140g)	2.7 4.2	¾ 1
Vegetables, stir-fried, takeaway	0.2	0	Tr	0.2	Tr	340g	0.7	¼

Vegetables and vegetable dishes

Although the dried vegetables in this list look like they contain a lot of sugar, this is only because the sugar is more concentrated when a food is dried – you will use much smaller amounts than you would for fresh, cooked or tinned vegetables.

Food name	Total sugars (g/100g)	Teaspoons (tsp) sugar/100g	Sucrose (g/100g)	Fructose (g/100g)	Glucose (g/100g)	Average portion size	Grams (g) sugar per average portion	Tsp sugar per average portion
Alfalfa sprouts, raw	0.3	0	Trace	0.2	0.1	1 cereal/ dessert bowl (80g)	0.2	0
Amaranth leaves, boiled in water	0.2	0	Tr	0.2	Tr	4 heaped tablespoons (80g)	0.2	0
Amaranth leaves, raw	0.2	0	Tr	0.2	Tr	1 cereal/ dessert bowl (80g)	0.2	0
Artichoke, globe, boiled, weighed as served	1.4	¼	1.7	1.6	1.5	2 globe hearts (80g)	1.1	¼
Artichoke, globe, raw	1.5	½	1.8	1.7	1.6	50g each	0.8	¼
Artichoke, Jerusalem, boiled in water, flesh only	1.6	½	1.9	1.8	1.7	3 heaped tablespoons (80g)	1.3	¼
Asparagus, boiled in water	1.4	¼	0.2	0.7	0.5	5 spears (80g)	1.1	¼
Asparagus, canned, re-heated, drained	1.0	¼	0.2	0.5	0.4	7 spears (80g)	0.8	¼
Asparagus, raw	1.9	½	0.1	1.1	0.7	5 spears (125g)	2.4	½
Aubergine, fried	2.6	¾	0.1	1.1	1.4	⅙ aubergine (80g)	2.1	½
Aubergine, raw	2.0	½	0.1	0.8	1.1	½ aubergine (130g)	2.6	¾
Aubergine, stuffed with lentils and vegetables	1.7	½	0.1	0.7	0.8	½ aubergine (280g)	4.8	1¼
Aubergine, stuffed with rice	6.0	1½	0.2	2.7	3.0	½ aubergine (280g)	16.8	4¼
Aubergine, stuffed with vegetables, cheese topping	3.2	¾	0.3	1.4	1.5	½ aubergine (280g)	9.0	2¼
Avocado, average, flesh only	0.5	¼	0.1	0.1	0.3	1 small (100g) 1 medium (145g) 1 large (195g)	0.5 0.7 1.0	¼ ¼ ¼
Bamboo shoots, canned, drained	0.7	¼	N	N	N	3 heaped tablespoons (80g)	0.6	¼
Beans, balor, canned, drained	1.6	½	N	N	N	3 heaped tablespoons (80g)	1.3	¼
Beans, broad, canned, re-heated, drained	0.6	¼	0.6	Tr	Tr	3 heaped tablespoons (80g)	0.5	¼
Beans, broad, frozen, boiled in water	1.3	¼	1.3	Tr	Tr	3 heaped tablespoons (80g)	1.0	¼
Beans, broad, whole, boiled in water	0.9	¼	0.6	0.2	0.1	3 heaped tablespoons (80g)	0.7	¼
Beans, broad, whole, raw	1.3	¼	0.9	0.3	0.1	2 tablespoons (120g)	1.6	½
Beans, cluster (guar), raw	2.9	¾	N	N	N	2 tablespoons (120g)	3.5	1

Food name	Total sugars (g/100g)	Teaspoons (tsp) sugar/100g	Sucrose (g/100g)	Fructose (g/100g)	Glucose (g/100g)	Average portion size	Grams (g) sugar per average portion	Tsp sugar per average portion
Beans, green, boiled in water	3.0	¾	0.5	1.2	1.3	4 heaped tablespoons (80g)	2.4	½
Beans, green/French, canned, re-heated, drained	1.0	¼	0.2	0.5	0.3	4 heaped tablespoons (80g)	0.8	¼
Beans, green/French, frozen, boiled in water	2.1	½	0.4	1.0	0.7	4 heaped tablespoons (80g)	1.7	½
Beans, green, raw	2.2	½	Tr	1.4	0.8	2 tablespoons (120g)	2.6	¾
Beans, papri, canned, drained	0.4	0	N	N	N	4 heaped tablespoons (80g)	0.3	0
Beans, papri, raw	1.8	½	N	N	N	2 tablespoons (120g)	2.2	½
Beans, runner, boiled in water	2.0	½	0.5	0.9	0.6	4 heaped tablespoons (80g)	1.6	½
Beans, runner, raw	2.8	¾	0.6	1.3	0.9	2 tablespoons (120g)	3.4	¾
Beans, valor, ends trimmed, raw	2.4	½	N	N	N	2 tablespoons (120g)	2.9	¾
Beansprouts, mung, boiled in water	1.4	¼	Tr	0.7	0.7	3 heaped tablespoon (80g)	1.1	¼
Beansprouts, mung, canned, drained	0.4	0	Tr	0.2	0.2	3 heaped tablespoons (80g)	0.3	0
Beansprouts, mung, raw	2.2	½	Tr	1.1	1.1	2 handfuls (80g)	1.8	½
Beansprouts, mung, stir-fried in oil	1.4	¼	Tr	0.8	0.6	3 heaped tablespoons (80g)	1.1	¼
Beetroot, boiled in water	8.8	2¼	8.5	0.1	0.2	3 'baby' whole or 7 slices (80g)	7.0	1¾
Beetroot, pickled, drained	5.6	1½	4.4	0.6	0.6	3 'baby' whole or 7 slices (80g)	4.5	1¼
Beetroot, raw	7.0	1¾	6.7	0.1	0.2	1 small whole (35g)	2.5	¾
Broccoli in cheese sauce, made with semi-skimmed milk, homemade	3.0	¾	Tr	0.7	0.4	main dish (200g) side dish (80g)	6.0 2.4	1½ ½
Broccoli in cheese sauce, made with skimmed milk, homemade	3.0	¾	Tr	0.7	0.4	main dish (200g) side dish (80g)	6.0 2.4	1½ ½
Broccoli in cheese sauce, made with whole milk, homemade	2.9	¾	Tr	0.7	0.4	main dish (200g) side dish (80g)	5.8 2.3	1½ ½
Broccoli, green, boiled in water	1.6	½	Tr	0.8	0.8	2 spears (80g)	1.3	¼

Food name	Total sugars (g/100g)	Teaspoons (tsp) sugar/100g	Sucrose (g/100g)	Fructose (g/100g)	Glucose (g/100g)	Average portion size	Grams (g) sugar per average portion	Tsp sugar per average portion
Broccoli, green, frozen, boiled in water	1.5	½	0.2	0.7	0.6	2 spears (80g)	1.2	¼
Broccoli, green, raw	1.9	½	Tr	1.2	0.7	2 spears (80g)	1.5	½
Broccoli, green, steamed	2.0	½	0.3	0.9	0.8	2 spears (80g)	1.6	½
Broccoli, purple sprouting, boiled in water	0.9	¼	0.1	0.5	0.3	2 spears (80g)	0.7	¼
Broccoli, purple sprouting, raw	2.1	½	0.3	1.1	0.7	2 spears (80g)	1.7	½
Brussels sprouts, boiled in water	3.0	¾	0.6	1.1	1.3	8 sprouts (80g)	2.4	½
Brussels sprouts, frozen, boiled in water	2.4	½	0.5	0.9	1.0	8 sprouts (80g)	1.9	½
Brussels sprouts, raw	3.1	¾	0.7	1.3	1.1	9 sprouts (90g)	2.8	¾
Bubble and squeak, homemade	1.6	½	0.3	0.6	0.7	200g	3.2	¾
Cabbage, average, boiled in water	2.8	¾	0.3	1.1	1.3	3 heaped tablespoons (80g)	2.2	½
Cabbage, average, raw	4.4	1	0.3	1.9	2.2	⅙ small cabbage or 2 handfuls sliced (80g)	3.5	1
Cabbage, Chinese, raw	1.4	¼	Tr	0.6	0.8	⅙ small cabbage or 2 handfuls sliced (80g)	1.1	¼
Cabbage, dried	37.1	9¼	2.7	16.3	18.1	2 tablespoons (80g)	29.7	7½
Cabbage, frozen, boiled in water	3.1	¾	0.6	1.2	1.3	3 heaped tablespoons (80g)	2.5	¾
Cabbage, green, boiled in water	2.3	½	0.4	0.9	1.0	3 heaped tablespoons (80g)	1.8	½
Cabbage, green, raw	4.1	1	0.3	1.8	2.0	⅙ small cabbage or 2 handfuls sliced (80g)	3.3	¾
Cabbage, red, boiled in water	2.0	½	0.2	0.9	0.9	3 heaped tablespoons (80g)	1.6	½
Cabbage, red, cooked with apple	7.5	2	3.9	2.1	1.6	3 heaped tablespoons (80g)	6.0	1½
Cabbage, red, raw	3.3	¾	0.4	1.4	1.5	⅙ small cabbage or 2 handfuls sliced (80g)	2.6	¾
Cabbage, white, boiled in water	3.2	¾	0.2	1.4	1.6	3 heaped tablespoons (80g)	2.6	¾
Cabbage, white, raw	4.8	1¼	0.3	2.1	2.4	⅙ small cabbage or 2 handfuls sliced (80g)	3.8	1

Food name	Total sugars (g/100g)	Teaspoons (tsp) sugar/100g	Sucrose (g/100g)	Fructose (g/100g)	Glucose (g/100g)	Average portion size	Grams (g) sugar per average portion	Tsp sugar per average portion
Carrots, frozen, boiled in water	3.3	¾	1.8	0.7	0.8	3 heaped tablespoons (80g)	2.6	¾
Carrots, old, boiled in water	5.5	1½	3.9	0.7	0.9	3 heaped tablespoons (80g)	4.4	1
Carrots, old, microwaved	7.2	1¾	5.0	1.1	1.1	3 heaped tablespoons (80g)	5.8	1½
Carrots, old, raw	7.2	1¾	5.0	1.1	1.1	⅓ cereal bowl, shredded (80g)	5.8	1½
Carrots, young, boiled in water	4.2	1	1.8	1.1	1.3	3 heaped tablespoons (80g)	3.4	¾
Carrots, young, canned in water, re-heated, drained	3.7	1	2.2	0.7	0.8	3 heaped tablespoons (80g)	3.0	¾
Carrots, young, raw	5.6	1½	2.4	1.5	1.7	⅓ cereal bowl, shredded (80g)	4.5	1¼
Cassava, baked	1.6	½	1.1	0.1	0.2	3 heaped tablespoons (80g)	1.3	¼
Cassava, boiled in water	1.4	¼	1.0	0.1	0.2	3 heaped tablespoons (80g)	1.1	¼
Cassava, frozen, raw	1.0	¼	0.7	0.1	0.1	3 heaped tablespoons (80g)	0.8	¼
Cassava, raw	1.5	½	1.1	0.1	0.2	¼ of a whole small tuber (1000g)	15.0	3¾
Cassava, steamed	1.5	½	1.1	0.1	0.2	3 heaped tablespoons (80g)	1.2	¼
Cauliflower cheese, made with semi-skimmed milk, homemade	3.2	¾	0.3	0.9	0.8	as a main dish (200g) as a side dish (90g)	6.4 2.9	1½ ¾
Cauliflower cheese, made with skimmed milk, homemade	3.2	¾	0.3	0.9	0.8	as a main dish (200g) as a side dish (90g)	6.4 3.0	1½ ¾
Cauliflower cheese, made with whole milk, homemade	3.1	¾	0.3	0.9	0.8	as a main dish (200g) as a side dish (90g)	6.2 2.8	1½ ¾
Cauliflower cheese, retail	1.9	½	0.1	0.5	0.6	1 whole 400g pack	7.6	2
Cauliflower, frozen, boiled in water	1.5	½	0.3	0.6	0.6	8 florets (80g)	1.2	¼
Cauliflower in white sauce, made with semi-skimmed milk, homemade	3.3	¾	0.3	0.7	0.6	main dish (200g) side dish (80g)	6.6 2.6	1¾ ¾

Food name	Total sugars (g/100g)	Teaspoons (tsp) sugar/100g	Sucrose (g/100g)	Fructose (g/100g)	Glucose (g/100g)	Average portion size	Grams (g) sugar per average portion	Tsp sugar per average
Cauliflower in white sauce, made with skimmed milk, homemade	3.3	¾	0.3	0.7	0.6	main dish (200g) side dish (80g)	6.6 2.7	1¾ ¾
Cauliflower in white sauce, made with whole milk, homemade	3.2	¾	0.3	0.7	0.6	main dish (200g) side dish (80g)	6.4 2.6	1½ ¾
Cauliflower, boiled in water	2.4	½	0.5	1.0	0.9	8 florets (80g)	1.9	½
Cauliflower, raw	2.9	¾	0.4	1.3	1.2	8 florets (80g)	2.3	½
Celeriac, boiled in water	1.5	½	1.0	0.3	0.2	3 heaped tablespoons (80g)	1.2	¼
Celeriac, raw	1.8	½	1.2	0.4	0.3	½ small (225g)	4.1	1
Celery, boiled in water	0.8	¼	0.2	0.3	0.3	3 heaped tablespoons (80g)	0.6	¼
Celery, raw	0.9	¼	0.2	0.3	0.4	3 sticks (80g)	0.7	¼
Chard, Swiss, boiled in water	0.4	0	Tr	0.2	0.2	3 heaped tablespoons (80g)	0.3	0
Chard, Swiss, raw	0.6	¼	Tr	0.2	0.4	½ small 200g pack (100g)	0.6	¼
Chicory, pale variety, boiled in water	0.5	¼	Tr	0.3	0.2	3 heaped tablespoons (80g)	0.4	0
Chicory, pale variety, raw	0.7	¼	Tr	0.4	0.3	1 whole chicory (85g)	0.6	¼
Cho cho fritters, fried in oil, homemade (West Indian dish)	2.9	¾	0.1	1.1	0.9	56g each	1.6	½
Cho cho, boiled in water	2.5	¾	Tr	1.3	1.1	3 heaped tablespoons (80g)	2.0	½
Cho cho, raw	3.1	¾	Tr	1.7	1.4	1 whole small gourd (200g) ½ large gourd (650g)	6.2 20.2	1½ 5
Cole (brassica) leaves, dried, boiled in water	0.9	¼	0.1	0.4	0.4	4 heaped tablespoons (80g)	0.7	¼
Courgette, boiled in water	1.9	½	0.2	0.9	0.8	3 heaped tablespoons (80g)	19.3	4¾
Courgette, dried	24.1	6	2.8	11.4	9.9	2 tablespoons (80g)	19.3	4¾
Courgette, fried	2.5	¾	0.3	1.2	1.0	3 heaped tablespoons (80g)	2.0	½
Courgette, raw	1.7	½	0.2	0.8	0.7	½ large courgette (80g)	1.4	¼
Cucumber, raw, flesh and skin	1.2	¼	0.0	0.7	0.5	2 inch piece (80g)	1.0	¼

Food name	Total sugars (g/100g)	Teaspoons (tsp) sugar/100g	Sucrose (g/100g)	Fructose (g/100g)	Glucose (g/100g)	Average portion size	Grams (g) sugar per average portion	Tsp sugar per average portion
Curly kale, boiled in water	0.9	¼	0.1	0.4	0.4	4 heaped tablespoons (80g)	0.7	¼
Curly kale, raw	1.3	¼	0.1	0.6	0.6	½ small 200g pack (100g)	1.3	¼
Endive, raw	1.0	¼	0.1	0.5	0.4	1 whole endive (85g)	0.9	¼
Fennel, Florence, boiled in water	1.4	¼	0.1	0.6	0.7	3 heaped tablespoons (80g)	1.1	¼
Fennel, Florence, raw	1.7	½	0.1	0.7	0.9	1 whole bulb (227g)	3.9	1
Garlic mushrooms, not coated, homemade	0.4	0	0.0	0.3	0.0	3 heaped tablespoons (80g)	0.3	0
Gherkins, raw	1.6	½	Tr	0.8	0.8	1 large (60g)	1.0	¼
Gourd, kantola, canned, drained	0.3	0	N	N	N	3 heaped tablespoons (80g)	0.2	0
Gourd, kantola, raw	0.9	¼	N	N	N	1 whole gourd (650g)	5.9	1½
Gourd, karela, canned, drained	0.2	0	N	N	N	3 heaped tablespoons (80g)	0.2	0
Gourd, karela, raw	Tr	0	Tr	Tr	Tr	½ karela (80g)	Tr	0
Gourd, ridge, raw	3.1	¾	Tr	1.6	1.5	1 whole gourd (118g)	3.7	1
Gourd, tinda, canned, drained	2.0	½	N	N	N	3 heaped tablespoons (80g)	1.6	½
Gourd, tinda, raw	2.8	¾	N	N	N	1 whole gourd (50g)	1.4	¼
Kohl rabi, boiled in water	3.0	¾	0.6	1.1	1.3	3 heaped tablespoons (80g)	2.4	½
Kohl rabi, raw	3.6	1	0.8	1.3	1.5	½ kohlrabi (75g)	2.7	¾
Laverbread	Tr	0	Tr	Tr	Tr	75g serving	Tr	0
Leeks in cheese sauce, made with semi-skimmed milk, homemade	2.6	¾	0.3	0.5	0.4	90g	2.3	½
Leeks in cheese sauce, made with skimmed milk, homemade	2.6	¾	0.3	0.5	0.4	90g	2.3	½
Leeks in cheese sauce, made with whole milk, homemade	2.5	¾	0.3	0.5	0.4	90g	2.3	½
Leeks, boiled in water	2.0	½	0.5	0.8	0.7	3 heaped tablespoons (80g)	1.6	½
Leeks, raw	2.2	½	0.5	0.9	0.8	1 leek (80g)	1.8	½

Food name

Food name	Total sugars (g/100g)	Teaspoons (tsp) sugar/100g	Sucrose (g/100g)	Fructose (g/100g)	Glucose (g/100g)	Average portion size	Grams (g) sugar per average portion	Tsp sugar per average portion
Lettuce, average, raw	1.4	¼	Tr	0.8	0.6	1 cereal/ dessert bowl (80g)	1.1	¼
Lotus tubers, raw	5.5	1½	N	N	N	1 large tuber (200g)	11.0	2¾
Marrow, boiled in water	1.4	¼	0.1	0.7	0.5	3 heaped tablespoons (80g)	1.1	¼
Marrow, parwal, canned, drained	0.4	0	N	N	N	3 heaped tablespoons (80g)	0.3	0
Marrow, parwal, raw	0.8	¼	N	N	N	65g	0.5	¼
Marrow, raw	2.1	½	0.2	1.1	0.8	65g	1.4	¼
Mushrooms, common, canned, re-heated, drained	Tr	0	Tr	Tr	Tr	14 button (80g)	Tr	0
Mushroom, dried	3.6	1	1.2	1.2	1.2	2 tablespoons (80g)	2.9	¾
Mushrooms, oyster, raw	Tr	0	Tr	Tr	Tr	3 handfuls slices (80g)	Tr	0
Mushrooms, straw, canned, drained	0.4	0	0.2	0.1	0.1	3 heaped tablespoons (80g)	0.3	0
Mushrooms, white, fried	0.4	0	Tr	0.4	Tr	3 heaped tablespoons (80g)	0.3	0
Mushrooms, white, raw	0.3	0	Tr	0.3	Tr	3 handfuls slices (80g)	0.2	0
Mushrooms, white, stewed in water	Tr	0	Tr	Tr	Tr	3 heaped tablespoons (80g)	Tr	0
Mustard and cress, raw	0.4	0	N	N	N	1 cereal/ dessert bowl (80g)	0.3	0
Mustard leaves, boiled in water	0.5	¼	Tr	0.2	0.3	4 heaped tablespoons (80g)	0.4	0
Mustard leaves, raw	0.8	¼	Tr	0.3	0.4	1 cereal/ dessert bowl (80g)	0.6	¼
Okra, boiled in water	2.3	½	0.9	0.8	0.6	3 heaped tablespoons (80g)	1.8	½
Okra, canned, drained	0.8	¼	0.3	0.3	0.2	3 heaped tablespoons (80g)	0.6	¼
Okra, raw	2.5	¾	0.9	0.9	0.6	16 medium (80g)	2.0	½
Okra, stir-fried in oil	3.6	1	1.4	1.3	0.9	3 heaped tablespoons (80g)	2.9	¾
Olives, green, in brine, drained, flesh and skin	Tr	0	Tr	Tr	Tr	3g each	0.0	0
Olives, green, in brine, drained, flesh and skin, weighed with stones	Tr	0	Tr	Tr	Tr	6g each	0.0	0

Food name	Total sugars (g/100g)	Teaspoons (tsp) sugar/100g	Sucrose (g/100g)	Fructose (g/100g)	Glucose (g/100g)	Average portion size	Grams (g) sugar per average portion	Tsp sugar per average portion
Onions, baked	7.7	2	2.6	2.2	2.9	1 medium onion (80g)	6.2	1½
Onions, boiled in water	4.2	1	1.4	1.2	1.6	3 heaped tablespoons (80g)	3.4	¾
Onions, dried, raw	54.4	13¾	18.4	15.8	20.2	2 tablespoons (80g)	43.5	11
Onions, fried	8.6	2¼	2.9	2.5	3.2	3 heaped tablespoons (80g)	6.9	1¾
Onions, pickled, cocktail/ silverskin, drained	2.2	½	0.2	1.3	0.7	2g each	0.0	0
Onions, pickled, drained	3.5	1	1.2	1.4	0.9	1 average (15g) each 1 large (25g) each	0.5 0.9	¼ ¼
Onions, raw	6.2	1½	2.1	1.8	2.3	1 medium onion (80g)	5.0	1¼
Pak choi, steamed	1.5	½	0.1	0.6	0.8	3 heaped tablespoons (80g)	1.2	¼
Parsnip, boiled in water	5.9	1½	4.5	0.5	0.8	3 heaped tablespoons (80g)	4.7	1¼
Parsnip, raw	5.7	1½	4.3	0.5	0.8	1 large (80g)	4.6	1¼
Pate, vegetable	0.2	0	Tr	0.2	Tr	75g	0.2	0
Patra leaves, raw	2.2	½	N	N	N	4 heaped tablespoons (80g)	1.8	½
Peas, boiled in water	1.2	¼	1.2	Tr	Tr	3 heaped tablespoons (80g)	1.0	¼
Peas, canned in water, re-heated, drained	1.7	½	1.7	Tr	Tr	3 heaped tablespoons (80g)	1.4	¼
Peas, dried, boiled in water	0.9	¼	0.8	Tr	Tr	3 heaped tablespoons (80g)	0.7	¼
Peas, frozen, microwaved	6.6	1¾	6.6	Tr	Tr	3 heaped tablespoons (80g)	5.3	1¼
Peas, frozen, raw	5.7	1½	5.7	Tr	Tr	1 tablespoon (30g)	1.7	½
Peas, mange-tout, boiled in water	2.8	¾	0.6	0.1	2.1	3 heaped tablespoons (80g)	2.2	½
Peas, mange-tout, raw	3.4	¾	0.5	0.3	2.6	1 handful (80g)	2.7	¾
Peas, mange-tout, stir-fried	3.3	¾	0.7	0.2	2.4	3 heaped tablespoons (80g)	2.6	¾
Peas, marrowfat, canned, re-heated, drained	0.9	¼	0.9	Tr	Tr	3 heaped tablespoons (80g)	0.7	¼
Peas, mushy, canned, re-heated	1.7	½	1.6	Tr	Tr	3 heaped tablespoons (80g)	1.4	¼

Food name	Total sugars (g/100g)	Teaspoons (tsp) sugar/100g	Sucrose (g/100g)	Fructose (g/100g)	Glucose (g/100g)	Average portion size	Grams (g) sugar per average portion	Tsp sugar per average portion
Peas, petit pois, canned, drained	2.4	½	2.4	Tr	Tr	3 heaped tablespoons (80g)	1.9	½
Peas, processed, canned, re-heated, drained	1.5	½	1.5	Tr	Tr	3 heaped tablespoons (80g)	1.2	¼
Peas, raw	2.3	½	2.1	0.1	0.1	1 tablespoon (30g)	0.7	¼
Peas, sugar-snap, boiled in water	3.4	¾	1.4	0.1	1.9	3 heaped tablespoons (80g)	2.7	¾
Peas, sugar-snap, raw	3.7	1	0.9	0.4	2.4	1 handful (80g)	3.0	¾
Pease pudding, canned, re-heated, drained	0.9	¼	0.9	Tr	Tr	3 heaped tablespoons (80g)	0.7	¼
Pepper, capsicum, red, boiled in water	3.3	¾	0.2	1.9	1.2	3 heaped tablespoons (80g)	2.6	¾
Pepper, capsicum, red, raw	4.2	1	Tr	2.2	2.0	½ pepper (80g)	3.4	¾
Pepper, capsicum, yellow, boiled in water	5.1	1¼	Tr	3.0	2.1	3 heaped tablespoons (80g)	4.1	1
Pepper, capsicum, yellow, raw	4.4	1	Tr	2.6	1.8	½ pepper (80g)	3.5	1
Peppers, capsicum, green, boiled in water	2.3	½	Tr	1.4	0.9	3 heaped tablespoons (80g)	1.8	½
Peppers, capsicum, green, raw	2.4	½	Tr	1.4	1.0	½ pepper (80g)	1.9	½
Plantain, boiled in water, flesh only	5.5	1½	3.9	0.9	0.8	3 heaped tablespoons (80g)	4.4	1
Plantain, green flesh, raw	5.7	1½	4.0	0.9	0.8	225g each	12.8	3¼
Plantain, ripe, fried	11.5	3	6.9	2.3	2.3	1 whole (200g)	23.0	5¾
Pumpkin, flesh only, boiled in water	1.8	½	0.4	0.6	0.7	3 heaped tablespoons (80g)	1.4	¼
Pumpkin, flesh only, raw	1.7	½	0.4	0.6	0.7	1 US cup (225g)	3.8	1
Raddiccio, raw	1.7	½	Tr	1.2	0.5	1 cereal/ dessert bowl (80g)	1.4	¼
Radish, red, raw, flesh and skin	1.9	½	Tr	0.7	1.2	10 radishes (80g)	1.5	½
Radish, white/mooli, raw	2.9	¾	0.2	1.3	1.4	3 heaped tablespoon (80g)	2.3	½
Rocket, raw	Tr	0	Tr	Tr	Tr	1 cereal/ dessert bowl (80g)	Tr	0
Roulade, spinach	2.0	½	0.2	0.1	0.1	1 thick slice (30g)	0.6	¼

Food name	Total sugars (g/100g)	Teaspoons (tsp) sugar/100g	Sucrose (g/100g)	Fructose (g/100g)	Glucose (g/100g)	Average portion size	Grams (g) sugar per average portion	Tsp sugar per average portion
Salsify, flesh only, boiled in water	1.4	¼	1.3	0.1	Tr	3 heaped tablespoons (80g)	1.1	¼
Salsify, flesh only, raw	1.5	½	1.4	0.1	Tr	200g	3.0	¾
Sauerkraut	1.1	¼	0.1	0.3	0.7	1 tablespoon (30g)	0.3	0
Seakale, stem only, boiled in water	0.6	¼	N	N	N	3 heaped tablespoons (80g)	0.5	¼
Seaweed, Irish moss, raw	Tr	0	Tr	Tr	Tr	35g	0.0	0
Seaweed, dried, raw	Tr	0	Tr	Tr	Tr	35g	0.0	0
Shallots, raw	3.3	¾	1.1	1.0	1.2	43g each	1.4	¼
Spinach, baby, boiled in water	Tr	0	Tr	Tr	Tr	2 heaped tablespoons (80g)	Tr	0
Spinach, baby, raw	Tr	0	Tr	Tr	Tr	1 cereal/ dessert bowl (80g)	Tr	0
Spinach, canned, drained	0.8	¼	0.3	0.3	0.3	2 heaped tablespoons (80g)	0.6	¼
Spinach, dried	12.9	3¼	4.3	4.3	4.3	2 heaped tablespoons (80g)	10.3	2½
Spinach, frozen, boiled in water	0.3	0	0.1	Tr	0.1	2 heaped tablespoons (80g)	0.2	0
Spinach, mature, boiled in water	0.8	¼	0.3	0.3	0.3	2 heaped tablespoons (80g)	0.6	¼
Spinach, mature, raw	1.5	½	0.5	0.5	0.5	1 cereal/ dessert bowl (80g)	1.2	¼
Spring greens, boiled in water	1.4	¼	0.1	0.6	0.7	4 heaped tablespoons (80g)	1.1	¼
Spring greens, raw	2.7	¾	0.2	1.2	1.3	1 cereal/ dessert bowl (80g)	2.2	½
Spring onions, bulbs and tops, raw	2.8	¾	0.2	1.4	1.2	8 onions (80g)	2.2	½
Squash, acorn, baked	1.6	½	0.2	0.9	0.5	3 heaped tablespoons (80g)	1.3	¼
Squash, acorn, raw	1.0	¼	0.1	0.6	0.3	½ medium squash (454g)	4.5	1¼
Squash, butternut, baked	3.9	1	1.3	1.3	1.3	3 heaped tablespoons (80g)	3.1	¾
Squash, butternut, raw	4.5	1¼	1.5	1.5	1.5	½ medium squash (454g)	20.4	5
Squash, spaghetti, baked	3.4	¾	0.8	1.2	1.4	3 heaped tablespoons (80g)	2.7	¾
Squash, spaghetti, raw	3.6	1	0.8	1.3	1.5	¼ medium squash (454g)	16.3	4

Food name	Total sugars (g/100g)	Teaspoons (tsp) sugar/100g	Sucrose (g/100g)	Fructose (g/100g)	Glucose (g/100g)	Average portion size	Grams (g) sugar per average portion	Tsp sugar per average portion
Swede, boiled in water, flesh only	2.2	½	0.1	0.9	1.2	3 heaped tablespoon (80g)	1.8	½
Swede, flesh only, raw	4.9	1¼	0.2	2.0	2.7	1/3 medium swede (320g)	15.7	4
Sweet potato, baked	14.5	3¾	N	N	N	3 heaped tablespoons (80g)	11.6	3
Sweet potato, boiled in water, flesh only	11.6	3	N	N	N	3 heaped tablespoons (80g)	9.3	2¼
Sweet potato, raw, flesh only	5.7	1½	4.4	0.6	0.7	1 large (80g)	4.6	1¼
Sweet potato, steamed	8.4	2	N	N	N	3 heaped tablespoons (80g)	6.7	1¾
Sweetcorn, baby, canned, drained	1.4	¼	Tr	0.4	1.0	6 baby corn (80g)	1.1	¼
Sweetcorn, baby, fresh and frozen, boiled in water	1.9	½	Tr	0.5	1.4	6 baby corn (80g)	1.5	½
Sweetcorn, dried	9.4	2¼	Tr	0.4	9.0	2 tablespoons (80g)	7.5	2
Sweetcorn, kernels, boiled 'on the cob' in water	2.5	¾	Tr	0.1	2.4	1 cob (80g)	2.0	½
Sweetcorn, kernels, boiled 'on the cob' in water, weighed with core	1.5	½	Tr	0.1	1.4	1 cob (350g)	5.3	1¼
Sweetcorn kernels, canned in water, drained	7.5	2	7.1	0.1	0.3	3 heaped tablespoons (80g)	6.0	1½
Sweetcorn, kernels, raw	2.0	½	Tr	0.1	1.9	3 heaped tablespoon (80g)	1.6	½
Tannia, raw	0.2	0	Tr	0.1	0.1	1 whole average corm (680g)	1.4	¼
Tapioca, raw	Tr	0	Tr	0.0	Tr	1 whole small 1lb tuber (454g)	Tr	0
Taro leaves, raw	2.2	½	N	N	N	2 handfuls shredded (80g)	1.8	½
Taro leaves, steamed	1.2	¼	N	N	N	3 heaped tablespoons (80g)	1.0	¼
Taro, baked	1.4	¼	0.9	0.2	0.2	3 heaped tablespoons (80g)	1.1	¼
Taro, boiled in water	0.9	¼	0.6	0.2	0.2	3 heaped tablespoons (80g)	0.7	¼
Taro, raw	1.1	¼	0.7	0.2	0.2	1 small 2 lb corm (907g)	9.8	2½

Sugar Counter

Food name	Total sugars (g/100g)	Teaspoons (tsp) sugar/100g	Sucrose (g/100g)	Fructose (g/100g)	Glucose (g/100g)	Average portion size	Grams (g) sugar per average portion	Tsp sugar per average portion
Taro, steamed	1.0	¼	0.7	0.2	0.2	3 heaped tablespoons (80g)	0.8	¼
Tigernuts	16.1	4	16.1	0.0	0.0	1 whole average tuber (260g)	41.9	10½
Tomatoes, canned, whole contents	3.8	1	Tr	1.9	1.9	2 plum tomatoes (80g)	3.0	¾
Tomatoes, cherry, raw	3.6	1	Tr	2.0	1.6	7 tomatoes (80g)	3.0	¾
Tomatoes, standard, fried	4.5	1¼	Tr	2.4	2.1	1 tomato (80g)	3.6	1
Tomatoes, standard, grilled, flesh and seeds only	3.4	¾	Tr	1.8	1.6	1 tomato (80g)	2.7	¾
Tomatoes, standard, raw	3.0	¾	Tr	1.6	1.4	1 tomato (80g)	2.4	½
Tomatoes, sun dried	2.9	¾	0.0	1.8	1.1	5 tomatoes (15g)	0.4	0
Turnip tops, boiled in water	0.1	0	Tr	Tr	0.1	4 heaped tablespoons (80g)	0.1	0
Turnip, boiled in water	1.9	½	0.3	0.7	0.9	3 heaped tablespoons (80g)	1.5	½
Turnip, flesh only, raw	4.5	1¼	0.6	1.7	2.3	1 whole small turnip (500g)	22.5	5¾
Vegetable puree	4.1	1	0.3	3.4	0.4	3 heaped tablespoons (80g)	3.3	1
Vegetable stir fry mix, fried in oil	3.9	1	1.1	1.2	1.4	3 heaped tablespoons (80g)	3.1	¾
Vegetables, mixed, canned, re-heated, drained	2.5	¾	0.7	0.9	0.9	3 heaped tablespoons (80g)	2.0	½
Vegetables, mixed, cooked with onion, spice and tomatoes, homemade	3.4	¾	0.6	1.4	1.4	3 heaped tablespoons (80g)	2.7	¾
Vegetables, mixed, frozen, boiled in water	3.6	1	2.8	0.4	0.4	3 heaped tablespoons (80g)	2.9	¾
Vegetables, mixed, pickled	3.3	¾	0.3	1.6	1.4	3 heaped tablespoons (80g)	2.6	¾
Vegetables, mixed, stir-fry type, frozen, fried in oil	3.9	1	1.1	1.2	1.4	3 heaped tablespoons (80g)	2.0	½
Vine leaves, preserved in brine	0.1	0	Tr	Tr	Tr	3 heaped tablespoons (80g)	0.1	0
Water chestnuts, canned, drained	3.4	¾	N	N	N	3 heaped tablespoons (80g)	2.7	¾
Water chestnuts, raw	4.8	1¼	N	N	N	8.5g each	0.4	0

Food name	Total sugars (g/100g)	Teaspoons (tsp) sugar/100g	Sucrose (g/100g)	Fructose (g/100g)	Glucose (g/100g)	Average portion size	Grams (g) sugar per average portion	Tsp sugar per average portion
Watercress, raw	0.4	0	0.1	0.1	0.2	1 cereal/ dessert bowl (80g)	0.3	0
Yam, baked	0.9	¼	0.5	0.1	0.3	3 heaped tablespoons (80g)	0.7	¼
Yam, boiled in water, flesh only	0.7	¼	0.4	0.1	0.2	3 heaped tablespoons (80g)	0.6	¼
Yam, flesh only, raw	0.7	¼	0.4	0.1	0.2	1 US cup cubed (136g)	1.0	¼
Yam, steamed	0.7	¼	0.4	0.1	0.2	3 heaped tablespoons (80g)	0.6	¼

Vegetarian dishes

Food name	Total sugars (g/100g)	Teaspoons (tsp) sugar/100g	Sucrose (g/100g)	Fructose (g/100g)	Glucose (g/100g)	Average portion size	Grams (g) sugar per average portion	Tsp sugar per average portion
Bean loaf, mixed beans, homemade	3.6	1	1.2	1.2	1.1	1 slice (126g)	4.5	1¼
Beanburger, aduki, fried in oil, homemade	2.3	½	1.0	0.5	0.7	240g each	5.5	1½
Beanburger, butter bean, fried in oil, homemade	3.0	¾	1.9	0.5	0.6	240g each	7.2	1¾
Beanburger, red kidney bean, fried in oil	2.6	¾	1.5	0.5	0.6	240g each	6.2	1½
Beanburger, soya, fried in oil	3.7	1	1.8	1.0	1.0	240g each	8.9	2¼
Callaloo and cho cho, homemade	2.2	½	0.5	0.9	0.9	370g	8.1	2
Callaloo and okra, homemade	1.9	½	0.5	0.7	0.7	370g	7.0	1¾
Casserole, bean and mixed vegetable, homemade	3.4	¾	1.8	0.8	0.8	small (180g) medium (260g) large (360g)	6.1 8.8 12.2	1½ 2¼ 3
Casserole, bean and root vegetable, homemade	3.2	¾	0.9	1.1	1.2	small (180g) medium (260g) large (360g)	5.7 8.3 11.5	1½ 2 3
Casserole, sweet potato and green banana, homemade (West Indian dish)	24.6	6¼	N	N	N	370g	91.0	22¾
Casserole, vegetable, homemade	5.1	1¼	2.1	1.4	1.6	small (180g) medium (260g) large (360g)	9.2 13.3 18.4	2¼ 3¼ 4½
Cauliflower with onions and chilli pepper, homemade (Bangladeshi dish)	3.3	¾	0.9	1.2	1.2	small (180g) medium (260g) large (360g)	5.9 8.6 11.9	1½ 2¼ 3
Chilli, bean and lentil, homemade	3.5	1	0.5	1.5	1.5	220g (no rice)	7.7	2
Chilli, Quorn, homemade	3.5	1	1.2	1.2	1.3	220g (no rice)	7.7	2
Chilli, vegetable, homemade	3.8	1	2.2	0.8	0.8	220g (no rice)	8.4	2
Chilli, vegetable, retail	2.4	½	0.7	0.9	0.8	390g	9.4	2¼
Courgettes with eggs, homemade (Greek dish)	2.0	½	0.3	0.9	0.8	370g	7.4	1¾

Food name	Total sugars (g/100g)	Teaspoons (tsp) sugar/100g	Sucrose (g/100g)	Fructose (g/100g)	Glucose (g/100g)	Average portion size	Grams (g) sugar per average portion	Tsp sugar per average portion
Crumble, vegetable, with tinned tomatoes, homemade	4.9	1¼	1.1	1.8	1.9	400g	19.6	5
Crumble, vegetable, with tinned tomatoes, wholemeal, homemade	5.0	1¼	1.2	1.8	1.9	400g	20.0	5
Crumble, vegetable, with white sauce, homemade	4.0	1	1.9	0.4	0.4	400g	16.0	4
Crumble, vegetable, with white sauce, wholemeal, homemade	4.6	1¼	2.3	0.5	0.5	400g	18.4	4½
Curry, almond, homemade	1.1	¼	0.8	0.1	0.1	3–4 tablespoons (200g)	2.2	½
Curry, bhindi subji, homemade	4.4	1	1.1	1.5	1.8	3–4 tablespoons (200g)	8.8	2¼
Curry, black gram, whole and red kidney bean, homemade	1.2	¼	0.5	0.3	0.4	3–4 tablespoons (200g)	2.4	½
Curry, black gram, whole, Bengali, homemade (thin consistency)	1.6	½	1.0	0.3	0.3	3–4 tablespoons (200g)	3.2	¾
Curry, black gram, whole, Gujerati, homemade (thick consistency)	2.5	¾	0.7	0.9	0.9	3–4 tablespoons (200g)	5.0	1¼
Curry, black-eye bean, homemade (Gujerati dish)	1.0	¼	0.8	0.1	0.1	3–4 tablespoons (200g)	2.0	½
Curry, black-eye bean, Punjabi, homemade	1.1	¼	0.7	0.1	0.2	3–4 tablespoons (200g)	2.2	½
Curry, Bombay potato, homemade	1.2	¼	0.3	0.4	0.5	3–4 tablespoons (200g)	2.4	½
Curry, cabbage, masala, homemade	6.4	1½	0.8	2.6	2.9	3–4 tablespoons (200g)	12.8	3¼
Curry, cauliflower and potato, homemade (Gujerati dish)	2.7	¾	0.6	1.1	1.3	3–4 tablespoons (200g)	5.4	1¼
Curry, chick pea dahl and spinach, homemade	0.9	¼	0.7	0.1	0.1	3–4 tablespoons (200g)	1.8	½

Food name	Total sugars (g/100g)	Teaspoons (tsp) sugar/100g	Sucrose (g/100g)	Fructose (g/100g)	Glucose (g/100g)	Average portion size	Grams (g) sugar per average portion	Tsp sugar per average portion
Curry, chick pea dhal, homemade (Punjabi dish)	1.9	½	1.0	0.5	0.4	3–4 tablespoons (200g)	3.8	1
Curry, chick pea, UK type, homemade	2.7	¾	0.9	0.9	0.9	3–4 tablespoons (200g)	5.4	1
Curry, chick pea, whole and potato, homemade (Gujerati dish containing natural yoghurt)	2.1	½	0.5	0.1	Tr	3–4 tablespoons (200g)	4.2	1
Curry, chick pea, whole and tomato, Gujerati, homemade	3.8	1	2.0	0.9	0.8	3–4 tablespoons (200g)	7.6	2
Curry, chick pea, whole and tomato, Punjabi, homemade	1.1	¼	0.7	0.2	0.2	3–4 tablespoons (200g)	2.2	½
Curry, chick pea, whole, Gujerati type, homemade	1.2	¼	1.1	0.1	Tr	3–4 tablespoons (200g)	2.4	½
Curry, courgette and potato, homemade (Punjabi dish)	1.8	½	0.1	0.9	0.8	3–4 tablespoons (200g)	3.6	1
Curry, gobi aloo sag, retail	3.3	¾	1.2	1.0	1.1	3–4 tablespoons (200g)	6.6	1¾
Curry, green bean, masala, homemade (Gujerati dish)	2.6	¾	1.1	0.9	0.6	3–4 tablespoons (200g)	5.2	1¼
Curry, karela, homemade (Punjabi dish)	3.3	¾	0.9	1.1	1.3	3–4 tablespoons (200g)	6.6	1¾
Curry, lentil, red/masoor dahl and mung bean dahl, homemade (thin consistency)	0.9	¼	0.5	0.2	0.2	3–4 tablespoons (200g)	1.8	½
Curry, lentil, red/masoor dahl and tomato, Punjabi, homemade (thick consistency)	2.4	½	0.5	1.0	0.9	3–4 tablespoons (200g)	4.8	1¼
Curry, lentil, red/masoor dahl and tomato, homemade (thin consistency)	1.1	¼	0.6	0.3	0.3	3–4 tablespoons (200g)	2.2	½

Food name	Total sugars (g/100g)	Teaspoons (tsp) sugar/100g	Sucrose (g/100g)	Fructose (g/100g)	Glucose (g/100g)	Average portion size	Grams (g) sugar per average portion	Tsp sugar per average portion
Curry, lentil, red/masoor dahl and vegetable, UK type, homemade	2.4	½	0.9	0.8	0.7	3–4 tablespoons (200g)	4.8	1¼
Curry, lentil, red/masoor dahl, mung bean dahl and tomato, homemade (Punjabi dish)	0.8	¼	0.3	0.2	0.2	3–4 tablespoons (200g)	1.6	½
Curry, lentil, red/masoor dahl, Punjabi, homemade (thick consistency)	3.9	1	1.7	1.0	1.2	3–4 tablespoons (200g)	7.8	2
Curry, lentil, red/masoor dahl, homemade (Bangladeshi dish, thin consistency)	2.2	½	1.1	0.5	0.6	3–4 tablespoons (200g)	4.4	1¼
Curry, lentil, whole/masoor, Gujerati, homemade (thick consistency)	3.1	¾	1.7	0.7	0.7	3–4 tablespoons (200g)	6.2	1½
Curry, lentil, whole/masoor, Punjabi, homemade (medium consistency)	1.4	¼	0.7	0.3	0.3	3–4 tablespoons (200g)	2.8	¾
Curry, mung bean dahl and spinach, homemade (Gujerati dish)	3.0	¾	2.1	0.5	0.4	3–4 tablespoons (200g)	6.0	1½
Curry, mung bean dahl and tomato, homemade (Punjabi dish)	0.8	¼	0.3	0.3	0.3	3–4 tablespoons (200g)	1.6	½
Curry, mung bean dahl, Bengali, homemade (thin consistency)	0.5	¼	0.2	0.1	0.1	3–4 tablespoons (200g)	1.0	¼
Curry, mung bean, whole and turnip leaves, homemade	0.3	0	0.1	0.0	0.1	3–4 tablespoons (200g)	0.6	¼
Curry, mung bean, whole, Gujerati, homemade (thick consistency)	2.5	¾	1.1	0.7	0.7	3–4 tablespoons (200g)	5.0	1¼
Curry, mung bean, whole, Punjabi, homemade (medium consistency)	1.0	¼	0.3	0.3	0.3	3–4 tablespoons (200g)	2.0	½

Food name	Total sugars (g/100g)	Teaspoons (tsp) sugar/100g	Sucrose (g/100g)	Fructose (g/100g)	Glucose (g/100g)	Average portion size	Grams (g) sugar per average portion	Tsp sugar per average portion
Curry, pea and potato, homemade	2.7	¾	1.5	0.5	0.6	3–4 tablespoons (200g)	5.4	1¼
Curry, pigeon pea dahl and tomato, homemade (thin consistency)	1.5	½	1.3	0.1	0.1	3–4 tablespoons (200g)	3.0	¾
Curry, pigeon pea dahl with tomatoes and peanuts, homemade (Gujerati dish)	1.0	¼	0.6	0.2	0.2	3–4 tablespoons (200g)	2.0	½
Curry, pigeon pea dahl, homemade	2.1	½	1.8	0.1	0.1	3–4 tablespoons (200g)	4.2	1
Curry, potato and pea, homemade (Bangladeshi dish)	3.7	1	1.7	0.9	1.0	3–4 tablespoons (200g)	7.4	1¾
Curry, potato, Gujerati, homemade	2.1	½	1.6	0.2	0.3	3–4 tablespoons (200g)	4.2	1
Curry, potato, Punjabi, homemade	2.4	½	0.6	0.8	0.9	3–4 tablespoons (200g)	4.8	1¼
Curry, red kidney and mung bean, whole, homemade	0.4	0	0.3	Tr	Tr	3–4 tablespoons (200g)	0.8	¼
Curry, red kidney bean, Gujerati, homemade (thin consistency)	2.3	½	1.7	0.3	0.3	3–4 tablespoons (200g)	4.6	1¼
Curry, red kidney bean, Punjabi, homemade (medium consistency)	1.2	¼	0.5	0.3	0.3	3–4 tablespoons (200g)	2.4	½
Curry, spinach and potato, masala, homemade	4.9	1¼	1.0	1.8	2.1	3–4 tablespoons (200g)	9.8	2½
Curry, tinda gourd and potato, homemade (Punjabi dish)	3.5	1	N	N	N	3–4 tablespoons (200g)	7.0	1¾
Curry, vegetable, frozen mixed vegetables, homemade	2.9	¾	1.8	0.5	0.6	3–4 tablespoons (200g)	5.8	1½
Curry, vegetable, in sweet sauce, UK type, homemade	3.9	1	0.8	1.6	1.5	3–4 tablespoons (200g)	7.8	2
Curry, vegetable, Islami, homemade	4.0	1	0.5	1.7	1.8	3–4 tablespoons (200g)	8.0	2

Food name	Total sugars (g/100g)	Teaspoons (tsp) sugar/100g	Sucrose (g/100g)	Fructose (g/100g)	Glucose (g/100g)	Average portion size	Grams (g) sugar per average portion	Tsp sugar per average portion
Curry, vegetable, Pakistani, homemade	3.9	1	1.3	1.2	1.3	3–4 tablespoons (200g)	7.8	2
Curry, vegetable, ready meal, without rice, cooked	3.4	¾	1.1	0.9	0.9	3–4 tablespoons (200g)	6.8	1¾
Curry, vegetable, retail, with rice	1.9	½	0.6	0.5	0.5	3–4 tablespoons (200g)	3.8	1
Curry, vegetable, West Indian, homemade	2.1	½	0.5	0.8	0.8	3–4 tablespoons (200g)	4.2	1
Curry, vegetable, with yogurt, UK type, homemade	4.0	1	0.8	1.1	1.2	3–4 tablespoons (200g)	8.0	2
Dosa, filling, vegetable, homemade	4.1	1	0.9	1.4	1.6	20g	0.8	¼
Dumplings, homemade	0.2	0	0.1	0.0	0.0	70g each	0.1	0
Khadhi (Gujerati dish)	4.5	1¼	1.2	Tr	Tr	370g	16.7	4¼
Khatiyu (Gujerati dish)	3.8	1	N	N	N	370g	14.1	3½
Khichadi	0.2	0	0.1	Tr	Tr	3–4 tablespoons (200g)	0.4	0
Lentil and nut roast, homemade	2.7	¾	N	N	N	1 slice (126g)	3.4	¾
Lentil and nut roast, with egg, homemade	2.6	¾	N	N	N	1 slice (126g)	3.3	¾
Lentil and potato pie, homemade	1.4	¼	0.7	0.3	0.4	160g	2.2	½
Lentil and rice roast, homemade	1.1	¼	0.6	0.2	0.3	160g	1.8	½
Lentil and rice roast, with egg, homemade	1.1	¼	0.6	0.2	0.3	160g	1.8	½
Lentil cutlets, homemade	1.2	¼	0.8	0.2	0.1	155g	1.9	½
Lentil pie, homemade	4.2	1	1.9	0.8	0.8	310g	13.0	3¼
Lentil roast, homemade	2.5	¾	N	N	N	128g	3.2	¾
Lentil roast, with egg, homemade	2.3	½	N	N	N	128g	2.9	¾
Mchicha, homemade (Tanzanian dish)	3.0	¾	0.9	1.0	1.1	370g	11.1	2¾
Methi aloo, homemade	1.5	½	0.2	0.7	0.6	360g	5.4	1¼

Food name	Total sugars (g/100g)	Teaspoons (tsp) sugar/100g	Sucrose (g/100g)	Fructose (g/100g)	Glucose (g/100g)	Average portion size	Grams (g) sugar per average portion	Tsp sugar per average portion
Moussaka, vegetable, homemade	2.4	½	0.4	0.6	0.7	325g	7.8	2
Moussaka, vegetable, retail	4.5	1¼	0.5	1.0	1.0	325g	14.6	3¾
Mushroom Dopiaza, retail	2.6	¾	0.7	0.9	1.0	3–4 tablespoons (200g)	5.2	1¼
Nut and rice roast, mixed nuts with egg, homemade	2.7	¾	N	N	N	1 thin slice (128g)	3.5	1
Nut and rice roast, mixed nuts, homemade	2.9	¾	N	N	N	1 thin slice (128g)	3.7	1
Nut and seed roast, mixed nuts and sunflower seeds with egg, homemade	2.7	¾	1.6	N	N	1 thin slice (128g)	3.5	1
Nut and seed roast, mixed nuts and sunflower seeds, homemade	2.9	¾	1.7	N	N	1 thin slice (128g)	3.7	1
Nut and vegetable roast, mixed nuts with egg, homemade	3.6	1	N	N	N	1 thin slice (128g)	4.6	1¼
Nut and vegetable roast, mixed nuts, homemade	3.8	1	N	N	N	1 thin slice (128g)	4.9	1¼
Nut croquettes, fried, homemade	2.5	¾	N	N	N	90g each	2.3	½
Nut cutlets, retail, fried	1.3	¼	0.7	0.2	0.3	155g	2.0	½
Nut cutlets, retail, grilled	1.4	¼	0.8	0.2	0.3	155g	2.2	½
Nut roast, homemade	4.1	1	2.8	0.4	0.4	128g	5.3	1¼
Nut roast, mixed nuts with egg, homemade	3.0	¾	N	N	N	128g	3.8	1
Nut, mushroom and rice roast, homemade	2.8	¾	N	N	N	128g	3.6	1
Okra with tomatoes and onion, Greek, homemade	4.2	1	1.2	1.6	1.4	250g	10.5	2¾
Okra with tomatoes and onion, West Indian, homemade	4.0	1	1.1	1.5	1.2	250g	10.0	2½

Food name	Total sugars (g/100g)	Teaspoons (tsp) sugar/100g	Sucrose (g/100g)	Fructose (g/100g)	Glucose (g/100g)	Average portion size	Grams (g) sugar per average portion	Tsp sugar per average portion
Pastries, Chinese, flaky (with bean and vegetable paste filling)	30.1	7½	N	N	N	small (60g) large (112g)	18.1 33.7	4½ 8½
Peppers, green, stuffed with rice, homemade	5.5	1½	0.1	2.8	2.6	1 whole stuffed pepper (350g)	19.3	4¾
Pie, cheese and potato, homemade	1.5	½	0.1	0.2	0.2	125g	1.9	½
Pie, lentil and cheese, homemade	1.5	½	0.8	0.4	0.4	125g	1.9	½
Pie, Quorn and vegetable	3.4	¾	1.1	0.2	0.4	155g	5.3	1¼
Pie, spinach, homemade	2.6	¾	0.4	0.6	0.5	155g	4.0	1
Pie, vegetable, homemade	2.8	¾	0.6	1.0	1.0	155g	4.3	1
Pie, vegetable, wholemeal, homemade	3.0	¾	0.7	1.0	1.0	155g	4.7	1¼
Potato, leek and celery bake	1.6	½	0.2	0.1	0.2	145g	2.3	½
Potatoes with onions and eggs, fried (Greek dish)	1.4	¼	0.5	0.4	0.5	190g	2.7	¾
Quorn korma	1.3	¼	0.6	0.3	0.3	3–4 tablespoons (200g)	2.6	¾
Ratatouille, homemade	3.3	¾	0.4	1.4	1.5	1 tablespoon (30g)	0.1	0
Ratatouille, retail	3.6	1	Tr	1.8	1.7	1 tablespoon (30g)	1.1	¼
Red pea loaf (West Indian dish)	0.9	¼	0.7	0.0	0.1	126g	1.1	¼
Saag, homemade	1.7	½	0.5	0.6	0.6	3–4 tablespoons (200g)	3.4	¾
Sambar, homemade	1.9	½	1.3	0.3	0.3	3–4 tablespoons (200g)	3.8	1
Shepherd's pie, vegetable (vegetable and lentil base with potato topping)	1.5	½	0.6	0.4	0.5	310g	4.7	1¼
Shepherd's pie, vegetable, retail (vegetable, lentil and barley base with potato topping)	1.7	½	0.5	0.5	0.6	310g	5.3	1¼

Food name	Total sugars (g/100g)	Teaspoons (tsp) sugar/100g	Sucrose (g/100g)	Fructose (g/100g)	Glucose (g/100g)	Average portion size	Grams (g) sugar per average portion	Tsp sugar per average portion
Sweet potato and onion layer (West Indian dish)	6.8	1¾	3.8	0.7	0.8	190g	12.9	3¼
Tinda subji, homemade	4.1	1	0.6	1.7	1.8	260g	10.7	2¾
Tomatoes, stuffed with rice (Greek dish)	7.7	2	1.7	2.9	2.9	350g	27.0	6¾
Tomatoes, stuffed with vegetables (sweetcorn, onion and mushroom stuffing)	7.4	1¾	2.9	2.2	2.2	350g	25.9	6½
Tori ki subji, homemade	3.9	1	0.5	1.7	1.7	3–4 tablespoons (200g)	7.8	2
Urad dahl, homemade	0.8	¼	0.3	0.3	0.2	260g	2.1	½
Vegeburger, retail, grilled	3.6	1	1.8	0.4	0.5	56g	2.0	½
Vegetable and cheese grill/burger, in crumbs, baked/grilled	1.3	¼	0.2	0.2	0.2	100g	1.3	¼
Vegetable bake, homemade	4.6	1¼	1.2	0.6	0.6	360g	16.6	4¼
Vegetable kiev, baked	1.3	¼	0.3	0.1	0.2	155g	2.0	½
Vine leaves, stuffed with rice (Greek dish)	10.5	2¾	0.9	4.6	5.0	4g each	0.4	0

Vegetarian meat alternatives

Food name	Total sugars (g/100g)	Teaspoons (tsp) sugar/100g	Sucrose (g/100g)	Fructose (g/100g)	Glucose (g/100g)	Average portion size	Grams (g) sugar per average portion	Tsp sugar per average portion
Quorn, pieces, as purchased	0.4	0	Tr	Tr	0.4	¼ 500g packet (125g)	0.5	¼
Sausages, vegetarian, baked/grilled	1.3	¼	0.2	0.5	0.5	2 sausages (80g)	1.0	¼
Soya mince, granules	5.4	1¼	5.4	0.1	Tr	1 50g packet	2.7	¾
Tempeh	0.9	¼	0.9	Tr	Tr	½ 200g packet (100g)	0.9	¼
Tempeh burgers, fried	1.0	¼	0.5	0.2	0.3	102g each	1.0	¼
Tofu burger, baked	2.6	¾	1.5	0.5	0.6	102g each	2.7	¾
Tofu spread	2.3	½	1.2	0.5	0.6	1 oz (28g)	0.6	¼
Tofu, soya bean, steamed	0.3	0	0.2	Tr	Tr	½ 300g carton (150g)	0.5	¼
Tofu, soya bean, steamed, fried	0.9	¼	0.6	0.1	0.1	½ 300g carton (150g)	1.4	¼
Vegebanger mix	3.3	¾	2.3	0.6	0.4	½ 150g packet (75g)	2.5	¾
Vegebanger mix, made up with water	1.2	¼	0.9	0.2	0.2	½ 150g packet (75g)	0.9	¼
Vegebanger mix, made up with water and egg	1.3	¼	0.9	0.2	0.2	½ 150g packet (75g)	1.0	¼
Vegebanger mix, made up with water and egg, fried	1.4	¼	1.0	0.3	0.2	½ 150g packet (75g)	1.0	¼
Vegebanger mix, made up with water and egg, fried	1.4	¼	1.0	0.3	0.2	½ 150g packet (75g)	1.1	¼
Vegebanger mix, made up with water, fried	1.4	¼	0.9	0.2	0.2	½ 150g packet (75g)	1.1	¼
Vegeburger mix	4.8	1¼	2.5	0.5	0.4	½ 150g packet (75g)	3.6	1
Vegeburger mix, made up with water	1.8	½	0.9	0.2	0.2	½ 150g packet (75g)	1.4	¼
Vegeburger mix, made up with water and egg	1.7	½	0.9	0.2	0.1	½ 150g packet (75g)	1.3	¼
Vegeburger mix, made up with water and egg, fried	1.8	½	0.9	0.2	0.2	½ 150g packet (75g)	1.4	¼
Vegeburger mix, made up with water and egg, grilled	1.9	½	1.0	0.2	0.2	½ 150g packet (75g)	1.4	¼
Vegeburger mix, made up with water, fried	1.9	½	1.0	0.2	0.2	½ 150g packet (75g)	1.4	¼
Vegeburger mix, made up with water, grilled	2.0	½	1.0	0.2	0.2	½ 150g packet (75g)	1.5	½
Vegeburger, retail, fried	3.4	¾	1.7	0.4	0.5	56g each	1.9	½